CANCER RELATED FATIGUE (CRF)

A comprehensive guide for patients
and healthcare providers

Dr. Bhratri Bhushan MD, DM

CONTENTS

Management of Fatigue

PREFACE

In the realm of oncology, fatigue often emerges as a silent yet profound symptom, impacting every facet of daily life. This book serves as a source of understanding and empowerment for those navigating the complex terrain of cancer-related fatigue (CRF). This book explores the multifaceted nature of CRF and offer practical strategies for managing this pervasive symptom. From pharmacological interventions to holistic approaches, each chapter delves into the nuances of CRF management, providing a comprehensive toolkit for survivors, caregivers, and healthcare professionals alike. As we journey together through these pages, may we find solace, support, and renewed hope on the path to reclaiming vitality and well-being.

CHAPTER 1: INTRODUCTION TO CANCER-RELATED FATIGUE

Cancer-related fatigue (CRF) is a complex and debilitating symptom experienced by many individuals undergoing cancer treatment or living with cancer. Unlike ordinary tiredness, CRF is pervasive, often unrelenting, and not entirely alleviated by rest. It can significantly impact a patient's quality of life, affecting their ability to engage in daily activities, work, and social interactions. Understanding and effectively managing CRF is essential for healthcare providers, patients, and caregivers alike.

Defining Cancer-Related Fatigue

Cancer-related fatigue (CRF) is a multifaceted and often misunderstood aspect of cancer and its treatment. Unlike regular tiredness, CRF is not alleviated by rest and can persist for extended periods, significantly impacting the quality of life of cancer patients.

Defining Cancer-Related Fatigue:

Cancer-related fatigue is commonly defined as an overwhelming and persistent sense of tiredness or exhaustion that is not proportional to recent activity and interferes with daily functioning. It is a subjective experience, varying greatly in severity and duration among individuals. CRF can occur at any stage of cancer treatment, from diagnosis through survivorship, and may persist for months or even years after treatment completion.

Prevalence of Cancer-Related Fatigue:

CRF is one of the most prevalent and distressing symptoms reported by cancer patients, affecting up to 80% of individuals undergoing treatment and approximately one-third of cancer survivors. Its prevalence varies depending on cancer type, treatment modality, and individual patient factors. For example, patients receiving chemotherapy or radiation therapy tend to experience higher levels of fatigue compared to those undergoing surgery alone.

Contributing Factors to Cancer-Related Fatigue:

The etiology of CRF is complex and multifactorial, involving biological, psychological, and social factors. Cancer and its treatment can directly contribute to fatigue through mechanisms such as inflammation, hormonal changes, anemia, and disruption of normal sleep-wake cycles. Additionally, psychological factors such as depression, anxiety, and distress can exacerbate fatigue, creating a vicious cycle of symptom burden.

Challenges in Managing Cancer-Related Fatigue:

Despite its prevalence and impact, CRF remains challenging to manage effectively. There is no one-size-fits-all approach to fatigue management, and interventions that work for one individual may not be effective for another. Furthermore, CRF often coexists with other cancer-related symptoms, such as pain, nausea, and depression, making it difficult to isolate and treat in isolation.

The Impact of Fatigue on Cancer Patients

Fatigue is a prevalent and debilitating symptom experienced by many cancer patients throughout their journey, influencing various aspects of their physical, emotional, and social well-being.

Physiological Manifestations of Fatigue:

Fatigue in cancer patients is often associated with a myriad of physiological changes, including alterations in inflammatory pathways, dysregulation of the hypothalamic-pituitary-adrenal axis, and disruption of sleep-wake cycles. These biological processes can contribute to feelings of exhaustion, weakness, and reduced stamina, making even simple tasks challenging for patients.

Psychological Implications of Fatigue:

Beyond its physical manifestations, fatigue can also take a toll on patients' psychological well-being.

3

Chronic fatigue is closely linked to symptoms of depression, anxiety, and decreased motivation, exacerbating the overall burden of the disease. Furthermore, the cyclical nature of fatigue, where rest does not necessarily alleviate symptoms, can lead to feelings of frustration, helplessness, and loss of control.

Effects on Daily Functioning:

Fatigue profoundly impacts the daily lives of cancer patients, limiting their ability to engage in routine activities such as work, household chores, and social interactions. Simple tasks that were once taken for granted become arduous challenges, leading to increased dependency on caregivers and diminished quality of life. Fatigue can also interfere with treatment adherence and compliance, potentially compromising treatment outcomes.

Implications for Treatment and Survivorship:

The presence of fatigue can significantly influence treatment decisions and outcomes in cancer patients. Severe fatigue may necessitate dose reductions or treatment delays, affecting the efficacy of therapy and overall prognosis. Moreover, persistent fatigue during survivorship can impair long-term functional status and hinder the process of rehabilitation and recovery.

Importance of Managing

Cancer-Related Fatigue

The impact of CRF extends far beyond mere physical exhaustion, affecting every facet of a patient's life. In this text, we explore the critical importance of effectively managing CRF, understanding its implications for treatment outcomes, quality of life, and overall well-being.

Understanding the Impact of Cancer-Related Fatigue:

CRF is characterized by a persistent and overwhelming sense of tiredness that is not alleviated by rest and can significantly impair a patient's ability to function on a daily basis. Its multifaceted nature influences not only physical well-being but also psychological and social aspects of a patient's life. Left unaddressed, CRF can lead to decreased treatment adherence, diminished quality of life, and increased healthcare utilization, posing significant challenges for both patients and healthcare providers.

Improving Treatment Tolerance and Outcomes:

Effective management of CRF is essential for optimizing treatment tolerance and outcomes in cancer patients. Fatigue can limit a patient's ability to tolerate aggressive treatment regimens, leading to dose reductions, treatment delays, or even discontinuation of therapy. By addressing CRF proactively, healthcare providers can help patients adhere to their prescribed treatment plans, thereby maximizing the likelihood of treatment success and improving long-term survival rates.

Enhancing Quality of Life:

Beyond its impact on treatment outcomes, managing CRF is crucial for enhancing the quality of life of cancer patients. Fatigue can profoundly affect a patient's ability to engage in activities of daily living, maintain employment, and participate in social and recreational pursuits. By alleviating fatigue symptoms, patients can regain a sense of control over their lives, experience improved mood and well-being, and reengage with the activities that bring them joy and fulfillment.

Supporting Survivorship and Long-Term Wellness:

The importance of managing CRF extends beyond the acute treatment phase, influencing long-term survivorship and overall wellness. Many cancer survivors continue to experience fatigue months or even years after completing treatment, underscoring the need for ongoing support and intervention. By addressing CRF during survivorship, healthcare providers can help survivors regain their strength and vitality, reduce the risk of disease recurrence, and promote long-term physical and emotional well-being.

CHAPTER 2: UNDERSTANDING THE CAUSES OF CANCER-RELATED FATIGUE

Cancer-related fatigue (CRF) arises from a complex interplay of biological, psychological, and social factors. Biologically, cancer and its treatments, such as chemotherapy, radiation, and surgery, can disrupt normal cellular function, leading to inflammation, hormonal imbalances, and anemia, all of which contribute to fatigue. Psychological factors, including stress, anxiety, and depression, often exacerbate fatigue by interfering with sleep and increasing overall emotional burden. Additionally, social factors such as isolation, changes in daily routine, and reduced physical activity can further intensify the sense of fatigue. Understanding these multifaceted causes is crucial for developing effective strategies to manage and alleviate CRF in cancer patients.

Biological Factors Contributing to Fatigue

Now we will explore the primary biological factors contributing to CRF, including inflammation, hormonal dysregulation, metabolic changes, anemia, and disruptions in the central nervous system.

Inflammation and Immune Response:

One of the key biological factors implicated in CRF is inflammation. Cancer and its treatments can trigger an inflammatory response, leading to the release of cytokines—proteins involved in cell signaling that regulate immune responses. Elevated levels of pro-inflammatory cytokines, such as interleukin-1 (IL-1), interleukin-6 (IL-6), and tumor necrosis factor-alpha (TNF-α), have been associated with increased fatigue. These cytokines can cross the blood-brain barrier and affect brain function, leading to symptoms of fatigue by altering neurotransmitter levels and disrupting normal brain activity.

Hormonal Dysregulation:

Cancer and its treatments can cause significant hormonal imbalances, contributing to fatigue. The hypothalamic-pituitary-adrenal (HPA) axis, which regulates stress responses and energy metabolism, can be disrupted by cancer-related processes. Abnormal cortisol levels, a key hormone produced by the adrenal glands, have been observed in patients with CRF. Cortisol plays a critical role in energy regulation, immune function, and the body's response to stress. Dysregulation of cortisol production can lead to persistent fatigue by impairing the body's ability to manage stress and maintain energy levels.

Metabolic Changes:

Cancer and its treatments can induce metabolic changes that contribute to fatigue. Alterations in energy production and utilization at the cellular level can lead to an energy deficit, causing feelings of exhaustion. Mitochondrial dysfunction, where the mitochondria—the cell's powerhouses—become less efficient at generating energy, has been implicated in CRF. Additionally, cancer treatments such as chemotherapy can disrupt normal metabolic processes, leading to muscle wasting and decreased physical strength, further exacerbating fatigue.

Anemia:

Anemia, characterized by a deficiency in red blood cells or hemoglobin, is a common condition in cancer patients and a significant contributor to CRF. Red blood cells are responsible for carrying oxygen to tissues and organs, and a deficiency can lead to reduced oxygen delivery, causing symptoms of fatigue and weakness. Chemotherapy and radiation therapy can damage bone marrow, where red blood cells are produced, leading to anemia. Additionally, cancer itself can interfere with red blood cell production through mechanisms such as bone marrow infiltration by tumor cells.

Central Nervous System Disruptions:

The central nervous system (CNS) plays a crucial role

in regulating energy levels and sleep-wake cycles. Cancer and its treatments can directly or indirectly affect the CNS, leading to fatigue. For example, neurotoxic effects of chemotherapy can cause cognitive impairments and disrupt normal brain function. Changes in neurotransmitter levels, such as serotonin and dopamine, which regulate mood and energy, have also been observed in patients with CRF. Disruptions in these neurotransmitter systems can lead to decreased motivation, increased perceived effort, and overall fatigue.

Psychological Roots of Cancer-Related Fatigue

While biological factors play a significant role in CRF, the psychological roots of this condition are equally important in understanding its full impact and developing effective management strategies.

Stress and Anxiety:

Stress and anxiety are prevalent among cancer patients due to the uncertainty and fear associated with a cancer diagnosis and treatment. The psychological stress of coping with cancer can activate the body's stress response, leading to the release of cortisol and other stress hormones. Chronic activation of this stress response can disrupt normal bodily functions and contribute to fatigue. Anxiety, characterized by excessive worry and fear, can further exacerbate fatigue by consuming mental energy and causing physical symptoms such as muscle tension and increased heart rate, which can be draining over time.

Depression:

Depression is a common comorbidity in cancer patients and is closely linked to CRF. Depression can manifest as a lack of energy, decreased motivation, and an overall sense of exhaustion. The overlap between symptoms of depression and CRF makes it challenging to distinguish between the two, but the presence of depression can significantly amplify the experience of fatigue. Biological changes associated with depression, such as alterations in neurotransmitter levels (e.g., serotonin and norepinephrine), can also contribute to the physical sensation of fatigue. Additionally, negative thought patterns and feelings of hopelessness associated with depression can drain psychological energy and lead to a sense of profound tiredness.

Sleep Disturbances:

Sleep disturbances are another significant psychological factor contributing to CRF. Many cancer patients experience insomnia, frequent awakenings, and poor sleep quality due to pain, anxiety, and the side effects of treatment. Poor sleep can lead to a vicious cycle where fatigue causes difficulty sleeping, and lack of sleep exacerbates fatigue. Psychological stress and worry about the illness can also interfere with the ability to fall and stay asleep. The resulting sleep deprivation impairs the body's ability to recover and regenerate, leading to increased fatigue during waking hours.

Cognitive Impairments:

Cognitive impairments, often referred to as "chemo brain," are common among cancer patients and can contribute to feelings of fatigue. These impairments can include difficulties with memory, attention, and executive functioning, making daily tasks more mentally taxing. The increased effort required to perform cognitive tasks can lead to mental exhaustion, which in turn contributes to overall fatigue. The psychological stress of coping with cognitive changes can also amplify feelings of fatigue, as patients may become frustrated and anxious about their cognitive abilities.

Emotional Burden:

The emotional burden of living with cancer can be overwhelming and is a significant psychological root of CRF. Cancer patients often experience a range of emotions, including fear, sadness, anger, and grief. Managing these intense emotions requires substantial psychological energy, which can contribute to overall feelings of fatigue. The emotional toll of frequent medical appointments, treatments, and the uncertainty of the future can also lead to chronic stress, further exacerbating fatigue.

Social Influences on Fatigue Experience

While biological and psychological factors play critical roles in the onset and persistence of CRF, social influences are equally significant in shaping the fatigue experience. Social factors such as support networks, socioeconomic status, cultural beliefs, and healthcare access can profoundly impact the severity and management of CRF.

The Role of Social Support:

One of the most significant social factors affecting CRF is the presence and quality of social support. Strong support networks, including family, friends, and healthcare providers, can provide emotional, practical, and informational support that helps alleviate fatigue. Emotional support can reduce feelings of isolation and stress, which are known contributors to fatigue. Practical support, such as assistance with daily activities and treatment logistics, can reduce the physical and mental burden on patients. Informational support, including guidance on managing symptoms and navigating the healthcare system, can empower patients and improve their overall well-being. Conversely, a lack of social support can exacerbate feelings of loneliness and helplessness, intensifying the experience of fatigue.

Socioeconomic Status and Its Impact:

Socioeconomic status (SES) is another critical social determinant of CRF. Patients with lower SES often face additional stressors, such as financial instability, lack of access to high-quality healthcare, and poor living conditions, all of which can contribute to fatigue. Financial strain can limit access to necessary treatments, medications, and supportive care services, leading to unmanaged symptoms and increased fatigue. Additionally, individuals with lower SES may have less flexibility to take time off work or seek assistance with household responsibilities, further compounding their fatigue. Addressing socioeconomic disparities is essential for providing equitable care and support to all cancer patients.

Cultural Beliefs and Practices:

Cultural beliefs and practices play a vital role in shaping how patients perceive and manage CRF. Different cultures have varying attitudes towards illness, fatigue, and seeking help. In some cultures, fatigue may be stigmatized or dismissed as a minor complaint, leading patients to underreport symptoms and forgo seeking necessary support. Cultural norms regarding stoicism and self-reliance can also prevent individuals from seeking assistance or expressing their struggles with fatigue. Healthcare providers must be culturally sensitive and aware of these dynamics to offer appropriate support and interventions that resonate with patients' cultural contexts.

Healthcare Access and Quality:

Access to high-quality healthcare is a crucial factor influencing the experience of CRF. Patients with limited access to healthcare services may not receive adequate symptom management, leading to untreated or poorly managed fatigue. Geographic barriers, such as living in rural or underserved areas, can limit access to specialized cancer care and supportive services. Additionally, disparities in healthcare quality, including provider expertise and availability of resources, can affect the management of CRF. Ensuring that all patients have access to comprehensive, high-quality care is essential for addressing CRF effectively.

The Impact of Work and Daily Life:

The demands of work and daily life can significantly influence the experience of CRF. Balancing employment, family responsibilities, and treatment can be overwhelming, leading to increased stress and fatigue. Patients who are unable to modify their work schedules or reduce their workload may experience higher levels of fatigue. Additionally, the lack of supportive workplace policies, such as flexible hours and medical leave, can exacerbate the impact of CRF on patients' lives. Supportive workplaces and policies that accommodate the needs of cancer patients can help mitigate fatigue and improve quality of life.

Social Isolation and Loneliness:

Social isolation and loneliness are significant contributors to CRF. The physical and emotional demands of cancer treatment can lead to reduced social interactions and withdrawal from previously enjoyed activities. This isolation can increase feelings of loneliness and depression, both of which are linked to heightened fatigue. Encouraging social engagement and providing opportunities for meaningful connections can help reduce feelings of isolation and improve patients' overall well-being.

CHAPTER 3: ASSESSMENT AND DIAGNOSIS OF CANCER-RELATED FATIGUE

Assessment and Diagnosis of Cancer-Related Fatigue: The assessment and diagnosis of cancer-related fatigue (CRF) are critical for providing effective management and improving patient outcomes. This process typically involves a comprehensive evaluation using both subjective and objective measures. Healthcare providers often rely on patient-reported outcomes, utilizing standardized questionnaires and scales to quantify fatigue severity, duration, and impact on daily activities. Additionally, a thorough medical history and physical examination are conducted to identify underlying causes and rule out other conditions contributing to fatigue. By accurately assessing and diagnosing CRF, healthcare professionals can tailor interventions to address this pervasive symptom and enhance the overall well-being of cancer patients.

Tools for Measuring Fatigue Levels

Accurate measurement of fatigue levels is essential for effective management and intervention. Various tools have been developed to quantify fatigue, encompassing subjective self-report questionnaires and objective performance-based assessments.

Subjective Self-Report Questionnaires:

Self-report questionnaires are the most commonly used tools for measuring fatigue due to their simplicity, ease of administration, and ability to capture the patient's personal experience. These tools rely on patients' perceptions of their fatigue severity, duration, and impact on daily life. Key questionnaires include:

1. The Brief Fatigue Inventory (BFI):
   - The BFI is a short, validated tool widely used in clinical settings to assess the severity of fatigue and its impact on daily functioning. It consists of nine items rated on a scale from 0 (no fatigue) to 10 (severe fatigue), addressing fatigue intensity at its worst, best, average, and currently, as well as the extent to which fatigue interferes with general activity, mood, walking ability, normal work, relations with others, and enjoyment of life. The BFI is quick to administer and provides a comprehensive overview of fatigue impact.

2. The Functional Assessment of Chronic Illness Therapy-Fatigue (FACIT-F):
   - The FACIT-F is a 13-item questionnaire specifically designed to measure fatigue in chronic illness populations, including cancer patients. It assesses fatigue intensity, functional limitations, and the emotional and social consequences of

fatigue. Patients rate each item on a scale from 0 (not at all) to 4 (very much), providing a detailed picture of the multidimensional nature of fatigue.

3. The Multidimensional Fatigue Inventory (MFI):

- The MFI is a 20-item self-report questionnaire that evaluates five dimensions of fatigue: general fatigue, physical fatigue, reduced activity, reduced motivation, and mental fatigue. Each item is rated on a scale from 1 (yes, that is true) to 5 (no, that is not true). The MFI's multidimensional approach allows for a nuanced understanding of fatigue's various aspects, making it useful for both clinical assessment and research studies.

Objective Performance-Based Assessments:

While self-report questionnaires provide valuable insights into patients 'subjective experiences of fatigue, objective performance-based assessments offer additional data on the physiological and functional aspects of fatigue. These tools include:

1. The Six-Minute Walk Test (6MWT):

- The 6MWT measures the distance a patient can walk in six minutes, providing an objective assessment of functional capacity and endurance. While primarily used to evaluate physical performance, it indirectly assesses fatigue by measuring the ability to sustain physical activity. It is particularly useful in clinical trials and rehabilitation settings to track changes in functional status over time.

2. Actigraphy:

- Actigraphy involves the use of wearable devices, such as wrist-worn accelerometers, to continuously monitor physical activity and sleep patterns. Actigraphy provides objective data on activity levels, rest-activity cycles, and sleep quality, offering insights into the behavioral manifestations of fatigue. This tool is especially valuable for capturing long-term patterns and variations in fatigue and activity levels.

3. Cognitive Performance Tests:

- Cognitive performance tests, such as the Psychomotor Vigilance Task (PVT) and the Trail Making Test (TMT), assess cognitive function and mental fatigue. These tests measure reaction time, attention, processing speed, and executive function, revealing the cognitive impact of fatigue. Cognitive performance tests are often used in conjunction with self-report questionnaires to provide a comprehensive assessment of fatigue's effects on both physical and mental domains.

Combined Approaches:

Combining subjective and objective measures provides a more comprehensive assessment of fatigue. This approach acknowledges the multifaceted nature of fatigue, capturing both patients' perceived experiences and observable functional impairments. Integrated assessment strategies can enhance the accuracy and reliability of fatigue measurement, guiding tailored interventions and improving patient outcomes.

How Healthcare Professionals Diagnose CRF

Given its complex nature, diagnosing CRF requires a comprehensive approach involving various assessment tools and clinical judgment. This text explores the methods healthcare professionals use to diagnose CRF, highlighting the importance of patient history, self-report questionnaires, physical examinations, and laboratory tests.

Understanding CRF:

CRF is characterized by an overwhelming sense of tiredness or exhaustion that is not proportional to recent activity and interferes with daily functioning. It can occur at any stage of cancer treatment, from diagnosis through survivorship, and may persist for months or even years after treatment completion. The multifactorial nature of CRF, involving biological, psychological, and social factors, necessitates a thorough and multifaceted diagnostic approach.

Patient History and Symptom Assessment:

The first step in diagnosing CRF is taking a detailed patient history and conducting a thorough symptom assessment. Healthcare professionals inquire about the onset, duration, and pattern of fatigue, as well as its impact on daily activities. They also explore other symptoms that may be associated with fatigue, such as pain, sleep disturbances, depression, and anxiety. Understanding the patient's medical history, including cancer type, stage, and treatment regimen, is crucial for identifying potential causes of fatigue.

1. Initial Consultation:

   - During the initial consultation, healthcare providers ask open-ended questions to encourage patients to describe their fatigue in their own words. Questions may include, "When did you first notice your fatigue?" "How does fatigue affect your daily life?" and "Are there specific activities that make your fatigue worse or better?"

2. Symptom Timeline:

   - Creating a symptom timeline helps clinicians identify patterns and potential triggers of fatigue. Patients are asked to describe the intensity and frequency of their fatigue over time, as well as any changes in their treatment or lifestyle that may have influenced their symptoms.

Self-Report Questionnaires:

Self-report questionnaires are essential tools for diagnosing CRF, providing standardized and quantifiable measures of fatigue severity, duration, and impact on quality of life. These questionnaires help healthcare professionals gather consistent data and compare results over time.

1. Brief Fatigue Inventory (BFI):

- The BFI is a widely used tool that assesses the severity of fatigue and its interference with daily activities. It consists of nine items rated on a scale from 0 (no fatigue) to 10 (severe fatigue), addressing fatigue intensity at its worst, best, average, and currently, as well as its impact on general activity, mood, walking ability, normal work, relations with others, and enjoyment of life.

2. Functional Assessment of Chronic Illness Therapy-Fatigue (FACIT-F):

- The FACIT-F is a 13-item questionnaire specifically designed to measure fatigue in chronic illness populations, including cancer patients. It assesses fatigue intensity, functional limitations, and the emotional and social consequences of fatigue. Patients rate each item on a scale from 0 (not at all) to 4 (very much).

3. Multidimensional Fatigue Inventory (MFI):

- The MFI evaluates five dimensions of fatigue: general fatigue, physical fatigue, reduced activity, reduced motivation, and mental fatigue. Each item is rated on a scale from 1 (yes, that is true) to 5 (no, that is not true). This multidimensional approach allows for a nuanced understanding of fatigue's various aspects.

Physical Examination:

A comprehensive physical examination is essential

for identifying potential physical causes of fatigue, such as anemia, infection, or thyroid dysfunction. During the examination, healthcare professionals assess the patient's overall physical condition, including vital signs, body weight, and muscle strength.

1. Vital Signs:
   - Monitoring vital signs, such as blood pressure, heart rate, and respiratory rate, helps identify any abnormalities that may contribute to fatigue. For example, tachycardia (rapid heart rate) can indicate anemia or dehydration, both of which can cause fatigue.

2. Body Weight and Nutritional Status:
   - Assessing body weight and nutritional status is important, as malnutrition or unintended weight loss can lead to fatigue. Healthcare professionals may conduct a dietary assessment to evaluate the patient's intake of essential nutrients.

3. Muscle Strength and Endurance:
   - Evaluating muscle strength and endurance can reveal physical deconditioning or muscle weakness, which are common contributors to fatigue. Simple tests, such as handgrip strength or the six-minute walk test, can provide valuable information about the patient's physical capacity.

Laboratory Tests and Diagnostic Imaging:

Laboratory tests and diagnostic imaging are used

to rule out medical conditions that may contribute to fatigue. These tests provide objective data on the patient's physiological status and help identify underlying issues that require treatment.

1. Complete Blood Count (CBC):
   - A CBC measures various components of the blood, including red and white blood cells and hemoglobin levels. Anemia, characterized by low hemoglobin levels, is a common cause of fatigue and can be detected through a CBC.

2. Thyroid Function Tests:
   - Thyroid function tests measure levels of thyroid hormones (T3 and T4) and thyroid-stimulating hormone (TSH). Hypothyroidism (underactive thyroid) can cause fatigue and is diagnosed through these tests.

3. Electrolyte Panel:
   - An electrolyte panel assesses levels of essential minerals, such as sodium, potassium, calcium, and magnesium. Imbalances in electrolytes can lead to fatigue and other symptoms.

4. Inflammatory Markers:
   - Tests for inflammatory markers, such as C-reactive protein (CRP) and erythrocyte sedimentation rate (ESR), can indicate the presence of inflammation, which is associated with fatigue.

5. Diagnostic Imaging:
   - Diagnostic imaging, such as chest X-rays or

CT scans, may be performed to detect infections, tumors, or other conditions that could contribute to fatigue.

Multidisciplinary Approach:

Diagnosing CRF often requires a multidisciplinary approach involving oncologists, primary care physicians, psychologists, and other healthcare professionals. Collaboration among specialists ensures a comprehensive evaluation of the patient's condition and facilitates the development of individualized treatment plans.

1. Oncologists:
   - Oncologists play a central role in diagnosing CRF, as they have detailed knowledge of the patient's cancer history and treatment regimen. They can identify potential treatment-related causes of fatigue and recommend appropriate interventions.

2. Primary Care Physicians:
   - Primary care physicians provide a holistic perspective on the patient's overall health and can identify comorbid conditions that may contribute to fatigue. They also coordinate care among various specialists.

3. Psychologists and Psychiatrists:
   - Mental health professionals assess the psychological aspects of fatigue, such as depression, anxiety, and stress. They can provide psychological interventions, such as cognitive-behavioral therapy

(CBT), to help manage fatigue.

4. Rehabilitation Specialists:
  - Physical therapists and occupational therapists assess physical functioning and develop exercise and rehabilitation programs to improve strength, endurance, and overall energy levels.

Patient-Reported Outcomes in Assessing Fatigue

Given its subjective nature, traditional clinical assessments alone are insufficient for capturing the full impact of CRF. Patient-reported outcomes (PROs) have emerged as vital tools in the assessment of fatigue, providing valuable insights into patients' experiences, perceptions, and the functional implications of fatigue on their daily lives.

Importance of Patient-Reported Outcomes:

PROs are essential for a comprehensive assessment of CRF as they directly reflect patients' experiences and perceptions. Unlike objective measures, which may not fully capture the subjective burden of fatigue, PROs provide a nuanced understanding of its severity, duration, and impact on physical, emotional, and social functioning. Incorporating PROs into clinical practice and research enhances the ability to tailor interventions to individual needs, ultimately improving patient care and outcomes.

1. Capturing the Subjective Experience:

- PROs allow patients to express their personal experiences of fatigue, including how it affects their daily activities, emotional well-being, and social interactions. This information is crucial for understanding the full scope of CRF and its impact on quality of life.

2. Individual Variability:

- Fatigue is a highly individual experience, varying widely among patients in terms of intensity, duration, and impact. PROs account for this variability by providing personalized data, enabling healthcare providers to develop customized management plans.

3. Monitoring Treatment Effects:

- PROs are invaluable for monitoring the effects of cancer treatments on fatigue levels. They help identify treatment-related fatigue and track changes over time, guiding adjustments to treatment plans and supportive care measures.

Methodologies for Assessing Fatigue Using PROs:

Various PRO instruments have been developed to assess fatigue in cancer patients. These tools range from single-item measures to comprehensive multidimensional questionnaires, each with its specific focus and application.

1. Single-Item Measures:

- Single-item measures, such as the Numeric

Rating Scale (NRS) for fatigue, ask patients to rate their fatigue intensity on a scale from 0 (no fatigue) to 10 (worst possible fatigue). While simple and easy to administer, these measures provide limited information and may not capture the multidimensional nature of fatigue.

2. Brief Fatigue Inventory (BFI):

- The BFI is a widely used PRO tool that assesses the severity of fatigue and its impact on daily functioning. It consists of nine items rated on a scale from 0 to 10, addressing fatigue intensity at its worst, best, average, and currently, as well as its interference with general activity, mood, walking ability, normal work, relations with others, and enjoyment of life.

3. Functional Assessment of Chronic Illness Therapy-Fatigue (FACIT-F):

- The FACIT-F is a 13-item questionnaire specifically designed to measure fatigue in chronic illness populations, including cancer patients. It assesses fatigue intensity, functional limitations, and the emotional and social consequences of fatigue. Patients rate each item on a scale from 0 (not at all) to 4 (very much), providing a detailed picture of the multidimensional nature of fatigue.

4. Multidimensional Fatigue Inventory (MFI):

- The MFI evaluates five dimensions of fatigue: general fatigue, physical fatigue, reduced activity, reduced motivation, and mental fatigue. Each item is rated on a scale from 1 (yes, that is true) to 5 (no, that is not true). This multidimensional approach allows for a nuanced understanding of fatigue's various aspects.

Benefits of Using PROs in Assessing CRF:

The use of PROs in assessing CRF offers several benefits, enhancing both clinical practice and research.

1. Enhanced Patient-Centered Care:
   - PROs place patients at the center of their care by valuing their subjective experiences. This approach fosters better communication between patients and healthcare providers, facilitating shared decision-making and personalized care.

2. Improved Symptom Management:
   - By providing detailed and individualized data on fatigue, PROs enable healthcare providers to identify specific areas of concern and tailor interventions accordingly. This targeted approach can lead to more effective symptom management and improved patient outcomes.

3. Research and Clinical Trials:
   - In research and clinical trials, PROs are essential for evaluating the impact of new treatments on fatigue. They provide robust data on the patient-reported efficacy and tolerability of interventions, contributing to evidence-based practice and the development of new therapies.

4. Longitudinal Monitoring:

- PROs allow for continuous monitoring of fatigue over time, helping to track changes and trends. This longitudinal data is crucial for understanding the trajectory of CRF and the long-term effects of cancer treatments.

Challenges in Using PROs:

Despite their benefits, the use of PROs in assessing CRF also presents several challenges.

1. Subjectivity and Bias:

- PROs are inherently subjective, and patients' responses may be influenced by various factors, such as mood, pain, or cognitive function. Ensuring the reliability and validity of PRO data requires careful consideration of these potential biases.

2. Patient Burden:

- Completing PRO questionnaires can be burdensome for some patients, particularly those experiencing severe fatigue or cognitive impairments. Simplifying PRO tools and providing adequate support for patients during the assessment process are essential for minimizing this burden.

3. Integration into Clinical Practice:

- Integrating PROs into routine clinical practice can be challenging due to time constraints, limited resources, and the need for appropriate training. Healthcare providers must be adequately trained to interpret PRO data and incorporate it into clinical decision-making effectively.

4. Standardization and Comparison:

 - The lack of standardization in PRO tools and scoring methods can complicate comparisons across studies and clinical settings. Developing standardized PRO measures and guidelines for their use is crucial for ensuring consistency and comparability of data.

CHAPTER 4: MANAGING CANCER-RELATED FATIGUE: MEDICAL APPROACHES

Managing cancer-related fatigue through medical approaches involves a combination of pharmacological treatments and supportive care strategies. Pharmacological treatments may include medications such as psychostimulants, antidepressants, and corticosteroids, which can help alleviate fatigue by addressing its underlying causes. Additionally, managing comorbid conditions like anemia or thyroid dysfunction with appropriate treatments is crucial. Supportive care strategies, such as nutritional support, pain management, and sleep hygiene, also play vital roles in mitigating fatigue. A personalized and comprehensive medical approach, tailored to the individual needs of each patient, can significantly improve the quality of life for those experiencing cancer-related fatigue.

Pharmacological Interventions for Fatigue

Managing CRF requires a multifaceted approach, including pharmacological interventions, which play a crucial role in alleviating fatigue.

The Nature of Cancer-Related Fatigue:

CRF is a multifactorial condition influenced by the cancer itself, treatment modalities (such as chemotherapy, radiation therapy, and surgery), and other comorbid conditions. Biological factors, including anemia, hormonal imbalances, and inflammatory cytokines, contribute to fatigue. Psychological factors like depression and anxiety, as well as social factors such as lack of support and socioeconomic status, also play significant roles. Understanding the complex nature of CRF is essential for developing effective pharmacological interventions.

Pharmacological Interventions for CRF:

Several classes of medications are used to manage CRF, each targeting different underlying mechanisms. These include psychostimulants, antidepressants, corticosteroids, and other supportive agents.

1. Psychostimulants:

Psychostimulants, such as methylphenidate and modafinil, are commonly used to manage CRF due to their ability to enhance alertness and reduce fatigue.

   - Methylphenidate:
   Methylphenidate, a central nervous system stimulant, is often prescribed to cancer

patients experiencing fatigue. It increases the levels of dopamine and norepinephrine in the brain, improving attention, concentration, and overall energy levels. Studies have shown that methylphenidate can significantly reduce fatigue in cancer patients, enhancing their quality of life. However, potential side effects include insomnia, increased heart rate, and anxiety, which need to be monitored closely.

- Modafinil:

Modafinil is another psychostimulant used to treat CRF, particularly in patients who experience excessive daytime sleepiness. It promotes wakefulness by modulating neurotransmitters involved in sleep-wake regulation. Clinical trials have demonstrated its efficacy in reducing fatigue and improving cognitive function in cancer patients. Common side effects include headache, nausea, and anxiety.

2. Antidepressants:

Antidepressants are used to manage CRF, especially when fatigue is associated with depression and anxiety. Selective serotonin reuptake inhibitors (SSRIs) and serotonin-norepinephrine reuptake inhibitors (SNRIs) are commonly prescribed.

- SSRIs (e.g., Fluoxetine, Sertraline):

SSRIs increase the levels of serotonin in the brain, which can help improve mood and reduce fatigue. They are particularly useful for patients with comorbid depression. While SSRIs are generally well-tolerated, side effects can include gastrointestinal disturbances, sexual dysfunction, and sleep disturbances.

- SNRIs (e.g., Venlafaxine, Duloxetine):
SNRIs enhance both serotonin and norepinephrine levels, addressing both mood and energy levels. They have been shown to be effective in reducing fatigue and improving quality of life in cancer patients. Potential side effects include nausea, dry mouth, and increased blood pressure.

3. Corticosteroids:

Corticosteroids, such as dexamethasone and prednisone, are used to manage CRF, particularly in patients with advanced cancer or those undergoing palliative care.

- Dexamethasone:
Dexamethasone is a potent anti-inflammatory and immunosuppressive agent that can reduce fatigue by decreasing inflammation and improving appetite and energy levels. It is often used in short courses to manage acute fatigue episodes. However, long-term use can lead to significant side effects, including immunosuppression, muscle weakness, and osteoporosis.

- Prednisone:
Prednisone is another corticosteroid used to manage fatigue in cancer patients. It shares similar

benefits and side effects with dexamethasone. The decision to use corticosteroids must balance the potential benefits with the risks of adverse effects.

4. Other Supportive Agents:

In addition to the above-mentioned medications, other supportive agents can be used to manage specific underlying causes of CRF.

- Erythropoiesis-Stimulating Agents (ESAs):

ESAs, such as erythropoietin and darbepoetin, are used to treat anemia-related fatigue in cancer patients. They stimulate red blood cell production, increasing oxygen delivery to tissues and reducing fatigue. However, their use is associated with risks such as thromboembolic events and hypertension, necessitating careful patient selection and monitoring.

- L-Carnitine:

L-Carnitine, a naturally occurring amino acid derivative, plays a role in energy production and has been studied for its potential to reduce fatigue in cancer patients. Some studies suggest that L-carnitine supplementation can improve fatigue and quality of life, but more research is needed to confirm its efficacy and safety.

- Ginseng:

Ginseng, an herbal supplement, has been investigated for its potential to alleviate fatigue. Some clinical trials have shown positive effects on reducing CRF, though the evidence is not yet conclusive. Potential side effects include insomnia and gastrointestinal disturbances.

Evaluating the Efficacy of Pharmacological Interventions:

The efficacy of pharmacological interventions for CRF varies depending on the patient population, type and stage of cancer, and the underlying causes of fatigue. Clinical trials and observational studies provide valuable insights into the effectiveness of these medications, but individual responses can differ. Therefore, a personalized approach is essential, taking into account the patient's specific circumstances, preferences, and overall health status.

Challenges and Considerations:

Several challenges and considerations must be addressed when using pharmacological interventions for CRF.

1. Balancing Benefits and Risks:
   - The potential benefits of pharmacological interventions must be weighed against their risks and side effects. For example, while psychostimulants can significantly reduce fatigue, they may cause insomnia and anxiety in some patients. Similarly, corticosteroids can improve energy levels but carry risks of long-term adverse effects.

2. Patient Selection:

- Careful patient selection is crucial for optimizing treatment outcomes. Factors such as the patient's medical history, comorbid conditions, and concurrent medications must be considered to minimize the risk of adverse effects and drug interactions.

3. Monitoring and Adjustments:

- Regular monitoring and follow-up are essential to assess the effectiveness of treatment and make necessary adjustments. This includes evaluating fatigue levels, monitoring for side effects, and adjusting dosages or switching medications as needed.

4. Integrating Non-Pharmacological Approaches:

- Pharmacological interventions should be integrated with non-pharmacological approaches, such as exercise, psychosocial support, and cognitive-behavioral therapy, to provide a comprehensive and holistic management plan for CRF.

Complementary Therapies
for Fatigue Management

Traditional treatments, such as pharmacological interventions and lifestyle modifications, play crucial roles in managing fatigue. However, complementary therapies offer additional options that can enhance symptom relief and improve overall well-being.

Understanding Complementary Therapies:

Complementary therapies, also known as integrative or alternative therapies, encompass a diverse range of approaches that complement conventional medical treatments. These therapies aim to promote holistic well-being by addressing the physical, emotional, and spiritual aspects of health. While not substitutes for standard medical care, complementary therapies can be valuable adjuncts in managing cancer-related symptoms, including fatigue.

1. Mind-Body Therapies:
   - Mind-body therapies, such as yoga, meditation, tai chi, and qigong, focus on the interconnectedness of mind, body, and spirit. These practices incorporate movement, breathing exercises, and mindfulness techniques to promote relaxation, reduce stress, and improve energy flow. Studies have shown that mind-body interventions can effectively reduce CRF and enhance overall quality of life in cancer patients and survivors.

2. Acupuncture:
   - Acupuncture is an ancient Chinese healing practice that involves inserting thin needles into specific points on the body to stimulate energy flow and promote balance. Acupuncture has been studied extensively for its effects on CRF, with evidence

suggesting that it can alleviate fatigue, improve sleep quality, and enhance overall well-being. The exact mechanisms underlying acupuncture's effects on fatigue are not fully understood but may involve modulation of neurotransmitters and neuroendocrine pathways.

3. Massage Therapy:

   - Massage therapy involves manipulating soft tissues of the body to promote relaxation, relieve muscle tension, and improve circulation. Several studies have demonstrated the efficacy of massage therapy in reducing CRF and improving quality of life in cancer patients. Massage may help alleviate physical symptoms associated with fatigue, such as muscle pain and stiffness, while also providing emotional support and promoting relaxation.

4. Nutritional Interventions:

   - Nutritional interventions focus on optimizing diet and nutritional status to support energy levels and overall well-being. Dietary modifications, such as increasing intake of nutrient-rich foods and staying hydrated, can help combat fatigue and improve energy levels. Specific dietary supplements, such as omega-3 fatty acids, vitamin D, and certain herbs, have been studied for their potential to alleviate CRF, though evidence is mixed and further research is needed.

5. Herbal Medicine and Supplements:

   - Herbal medicine and dietary supplements, such

as ginseng, ashwagandha, and coenzyme Q10, have been explored for their potential to reduce CRF and improve energy levels. While some studies suggest benefits, the evidence supporting the use of herbal remedies and supplements for fatigue management is limited, and safety concerns exist regarding potential interactions with medications and variability in product quality.

6. Energy-Based Therapies:

-   Energy-based therapies, such as Reiki, therapeutic touch, and healing touch, focus on balancing the body's energy fields to promote relaxation, reduce stress, and support healing. While the mechanisms of action are not well understood, these therapies are believed to influence the body's bioenergetic fields and may have beneficial effects on CRF and overall well-being. Research in this area is ongoing, with promising but inconclusive results.

Integrating Complementary Therapies into Fatigue Management:

Integrating complementary therapies into comprehensive fatigue management plans requires a personalized and multidisciplinary approach. Healthcare providers should consider individual patient preferences, beliefs, and values when recommending complementary therapies. Collaboration between conventional and complementary healthcare providers is essential to ensure safe and effective integration of therapies and to monitor for potential interactions and adverse effects.

Considerations for Integration:

1. Evidence-Based Practice:

- Healthcare providers should prioritize evidence-based complementary therapies supported by scientific research. While some therapies have demonstrated efficacy in reducing CRF, others may lack sufficient evidence or pose safety concerns. Patients should be informed of the potential benefits, risks, and limitations of each therapy to make informed decisions.

2. Safety and Monitoring:

- Safety considerations are paramount when integrating complementary therapies into fatigue management plans. Patients should be screened for contraindications and potential interactions with conventional treatments. Regular monitoring and communication between healthcare providers and patients are essential to ensure safety and detect any adverse effects promptly.

3. Patient Education and Empowerment:

- Patient education plays a crucial role in facilitating informed decision-making and empowering patients to actively participate in their care. Healthcare providers should provide accurate information about complementary therapies, including their mechanisms, potential benefits, and limitations. Patients should also be encouraged to communicate openly about their experiences, preferences, and concerns.

4. Holistic Approach:

- Integrating complementary therapies into fatigue management requires a holistic approach that addresses the physical, emotional, and spiritual aspects of health. Healthcare providers should consider the unique needs and preferences of each patient and tailor treatment plans accordingly. Combining complementary therapies with conventional treatments and supportive care measures can optimize outcomes and enhance overall well-being.

Energy Conservation Techniques

Energy conservation techniques (ECTs) are practical strategies designed to help individuals manage fatigue and conserve their energy for essential activities. By adopting ECTs, cancer patients can optimize their energy levels, reduce fatigue-related distress, and maintain a sense of independence and autonomy.

Understanding Energy Conservation:

Energy conservation involves prioritizing activities, pacing oneself, and making conscious efforts to reduce unnecessary physical and mental exertion. The goal of energy conservation is to maximize energy levels for essential tasks while minimizing fatigue-related symptoms and functional limitations. This approach recognizes the finite nature of energy reserves and emphasizes the importance of self-awareness, planning, and adaptation.

Principles of Energy Conservation:

1. Pacing:
   - Pacing involves breaking tasks into manageable segments and alternating periods of activity with rest. By pacing oneself, individuals can avoid overexertion and prevent depletion of energy reserves. It is essential to listen to the body's signals and take breaks as needed to prevent fatigue from escalating.

2. Prioritization:
   - Prioritization involves identifying and focusing on essential tasks while delegating or postponing non-essential activities. By setting priorities, individuals can conserve energy for activities that are most important to them, such as self-care, work, and spending time with loved ones.

3. Simplification:
   - Simplification involves finding ways to streamline tasks and reduce unnecessary physical and cognitive demands. This may include using assistive devices, delegating responsibilities, and organizing the environment for efficiency.

Simplifying tasks can help conserve energy and minimize fatigue-related stress.

4. Optimization:

- Optimization involves identifying and implementing strategies to perform tasks more efficiently and effectively. This may include using ergonomic principles, modifying workstations, and adopting energy-saving techniques. By optimizing task performance, individuals can achieve their goals with minimal expenditure of energy.

Energy Conservation Techniques:

1. Activity Planning:

- Planning activities in advance allows individuals to allocate their energy resources strategically. Breaking tasks into smaller steps, setting realistic goals, and scheduling rest breaks can help prevent fatigue and promote productivity. It is essential to prioritize activities based on importance and energy requirements.

2. Pacing and Rest Breaks:

- Pacing involves balancing activity and rest to prevent overexertion and conserve energy. Individuals can pace themselves by alternating between periods of activity and rest, taking short breaks between tasks, and listening to their body's signals. Scheduled rest breaks can help prevent fatigue from escalating and promote recovery.

3. Energy-Saving Strategies:

- Energy-saving strategies involve optimizing task performance to minimize energy expenditure. This may include using assistive devices, delegating tasks, and simplifying routines. By adopting energy-saving techniques, individuals can conserve energy for essential activities and reduce fatigue-related strain.

4. Work Simplification:
-   Work simplification techniques involve breaking tasks into manageable steps, organizing the environment for efficiency, and reducing unnecessary physical and cognitive demands. This may include decluttering workspaces, using ergonomic tools, and prioritizing tasks based on importance and energy requirements. Simplifying work tasks can help prevent fatigue and improve productivity.

5. Adaptive Equipment and Assistive Devices:
- Adaptive equipment and assistive devices can help individuals conserve energy and perform tasks more independently. This may include mobility aids, adaptive utensils, and ergonomic furniture. By using assistive devices, individuals can reduce physical exertion and maintain their functional independence.

6. Mindfulness and Stress Reduction:
- Mindfulness techniques, such as deep breathing, meditation, and progressive muscle relaxation, can help individuals manage stress and conserve energy.

By practicing mindfulness, individuals can reduce mental and emotional fatigue, promote relaxation, and improve overall well-being.

Benefits of Energy Conservation Techniques:

1. Improved Energy Levels:
   - Energy conservation techniques help individuals optimize their energy levels and prevent fatigue-related exhaustion. By pacing themselves, prioritizing activities, and using energy-saving strategies, individuals can conserve energy for essential tasks and maintain their functional independence.

2. Enhanced Quality of Life:
   - Energy conservation techniques can improve quality of life by reducing fatigue-related distress and functional limitations. By adopting practical strategies to manage CRF, individuals can remain engaged in meaningful activities, maintain social connections, and preserve their sense of identity and autonomy.

3. Increased Independence:
   - Energy conservation techniques empower individuals to take control of their fatigue and manage their symptoms more effectively. By incorporating ECTs into daily life, individuals can increase their independence and autonomy, reduce reliance on others for assistance, and maintain a sense of self-efficacy and empowerment.

4. Better Disease Management:

- Energy conservation techniques complement conventional treatments and supportive care measures for managing CRF. By incorporating ECTs into comprehensive fatigue management plans, healthcare providers can enhance treatment outcomes, improve patient adherence, and promote overall well-being.

Considerations for Implementation:

1. Individualization:

- Energy conservation techniques should be tailored to the individual needs, preferences, and circumstances of each patient. Healthcare providers should work collaboratively with patients to identify strategies that are feasible, acceptable, and effective for managing CRF.

2. Education and Training:

- Education and training are essential for empowering individuals to implement energy conservation techniques effectively. Healthcare providers should provide guidance on pacing, prioritization, and energy-saving strategies, as well as practical tips for integrating ECTs into daily life.

3. Multidisciplinary Collaboration:

- Multidisciplinary collaboration is key to successful implementation of energy conservation techniques. Healthcare providers, including physicians, nurses, occupational therapists, and physical therapists, should work together to develop individualized fatigue management plans that incorporate ECTs and address the unique needs of each patient.

4. Monitoring and Evaluation:

- Monitoring and evaluation are essential for assessing the effectiveness of energy conservation techniques and making necessary adjustments. Healthcare providers should regularly assess fatigue levels, functional status, and adherence to ECTs, as well as provide ongoing support and encouragement to patients.

CHAPTER 5: MANAGING CANCER-RELATED FATIGUE: LIFESTYLE AND SELF-CARE

Managing cancer-related fatigue through lifestyle and self-care strategies involves adopting healthy habits and making conscious choices to support overall well-being. Regular physical activity, such as walking, gentle stretching, or yoga, can help improve energy levels and reduce fatigue. Adequate nutrition, including a balanced diet rich in fruits, vegetables, lean proteins, and whole grains, provides essential nutrients to support energy production and maintain strength. Prioritizing sleep hygiene practices, such as maintaining a consistent sleep schedule and creating a relaxing bedtime routine, can enhance restorative sleep and combat fatigue. Additionally, managing stress through relaxation techniques, mindfulness, and social support can help alleviate fatigue-related distress and promote emotional well-being. By incorporating these lifestyle and self-care strategies into daily life, cancer patients can effectively manage fatigue and improve their quality of life.

Nutrition and Exercise Strategies

While there is no single solution for managing

CRF, adopting healthy lifestyle habits, including nutrition and exercise strategies, can play a crucial role in mitigating fatigue and improving overall well-being.

Nutrition Strategies:

1. Balanced Diet:
   - Consuming a balanced diet rich in fruits, vegetables, whole grains, lean proteins, and healthy fats provides essential nutrients to support overall health and energy levels. Nutrient-dense foods can help combat fatigue and maintain strength during cancer treatment and recovery.

2. Hydration:
   - Staying hydrated is essential for preventing dehydration and maintaining energy levels. Cancer patients should aim to drink an adequate amount of fluids throughout the day, choosing water, herbal teas, and electrolyte-rich beverages over sugary or caffeinated drinks.

3. Small, Frequent Meals:
   - Eating small, frequent meals and snacks throughout the day can help stabilize blood sugar levels and prevent energy crashes. Opting for nutrient-dense snacks, such as nuts, seeds, yogurt, and fresh fruit, can provide sustained energy and combat fatigue.

4. Protein-Rich Foods:
   - Including protein-rich foods, such as lean meats,

poultry, fish, eggs, dairy products, legumes, and tofu, in meals and snacks can help support muscle strength and repair during cancer treatment and recovery.

5. Supplementation:

- In some cases, cancer patients may require nutritional supplementation to address specific deficiencies or support energy levels. Healthcare providers may recommend supplements such as vitamin D, vitamin B12, iron, and omega-3 fatty acids based on individual needs and treatment-related factors.

Exercise Strategies:

1. Low-Intensity Exercise:

- Engaging in low-intensity exercises, such as walking, cycling, swimming, or gentle yoga, can help improve energy levels and reduce fatigue in cancer patients. These activities promote circulation, oxygenation, and muscle strength without causing excessive exertion.

2. Pacing and Rest:

- Pacing oneself and incorporating rest breaks into exercise routines are essential for preventing overexertion and conserving energy. Cancer patients should listen to their bodies and adjust the intensity and duration of exercise based on how they feel.

3. Progressive Exercise:

- Gradually increasing the duration, frequency, and intensity of exercise over time can help build stamina and endurance in cancer patients. Progressive exercise programs should be tailored to individual fitness levels, treatment regimens, and health status.

4. Resistance Training:

- Incorporating resistance training exercises, such as weightlifting, resistance bands, or bodyweight exercises, can help maintain muscle mass and strength during cancer treatment and recovery. Resistance training also improves bone health and functional capacity.

5. Flexibility and Balance Exercises:

- Practicing flexibility and balance exercises, such as stretching, Pilates, or tai chi, can enhance mobility, coordination, and overall well-being in cancer patients. These activities promote relaxation, reduce muscle tension, and improve posture.

Benefits of Nutrition and Exercise:

1. Improved Energy Levels:

- Nutrition and exercise strategies help improve energy levels and combat fatigue in cancer patients. Nutrient-dense foods provide essential fuel for the body, while regular physical activity promotes circulation, oxygenation, and muscle strength.

2. Enhanced Physical Functioning:

- Engaging in regular exercise helps maintain

muscle mass, strength, and flexibility, reducing the risk of functional decline and disability in cancer patients. Proper nutrition supports optimal physical functioning and supports the body's healing and recovery processes.

3. Emotional Well-Being:

- Nutrition and exercise have positive effects on mental health and emotional well-being. Physical activity releases endorphins, neurotransmitters that promote feelings of happiness and relaxation, while nutritious foods provide essential nutrients for brain health and mood regulation.

4. Supportive Care:

- Nutrition and exercise are integral components of supportive care for cancer patients, complementing medical treatments and improving overall quality of life. These strategies empower patients to take an active role in their health and well-being during cancer treatment and recovery.

Considerations for Implementation:

1. Individualization:

- Nutrition and exercise strategies should be tailored to the individual needs, preferences, and circumstances of each cancer patient. Healthcare providers should consider factors such as treatment regimens, side effects, comorbidities, and functional status when designing personalized nutrition and exercise plans.

2. Safety and Monitoring:

- Cancer patients should consult with their healthcare providers before starting any new nutrition or exercise regimen, especially during active treatment. Regular monitoring and communication with healthcare providers are essential for ensuring safety, optimizing outcomes, and addressing any concerns or complications.

3. Gradual Progression:

- Cancer patients should start slowly and gradually progress with nutrition and exercise programs, listening to their bodies and adjusting activities based on how they feel. Overexertion and fatigue should be avoided, and rest breaks should be incorporated as needed.

4. Multidisciplinary Collaboration:

- Multidisciplinary collaboration among healthcare providers, including physicians, dietitians, exercise physiologists, physical therapists, and oncology nurses, is essential for comprehensive fatigue management. Collaborative care ensures that patients receive integrated, holistic support that addresses their unique needs and circumstances.

Pacing Activities and Goal Setting

Pacing activities and goal setting are two essential

strategies for managing CRF, enabling individuals to conserve energy, prevent overexertion, and maintain a sense of control and accomplishment. Lets explore the principles of pacing and goal setting in fatigue management, discussing their benefits, implementation strategies, and considerations for cancer patients and survivors.

Understanding Pacing Activities:

Pacing activities involves breaking tasks into manageable segments, alternating periods of activity with rest, and listening to the body's signals to prevent overexertion and conserve energy. The goal of pacing is to maintain a balance between activity and rest, allowing individuals to accomplish their goals without exacerbating fatigue or functional limitations. Pacing activities promotes self-awareness, adaptability, and empowerment, empowering individuals to take an active role in managing their fatigue.

Principles of Pacing:

1. Break Tasks into Smaller Steps:
   - Breaking tasks into smaller, more manageable steps reduces the cognitive and physical demands of activities, making them easier to accomplish without excessive exertion. By dividing tasks into manageable segments, individuals can pace themselves more effectively and prevent fatigue-related exhaustion.

2. Alternate Activity with Rest:

- Alternating periods of activity with rest allows individuals to conserve energy and prevent overexertion. Short breaks between tasks provide opportunities for relaxation, rejuvenation, and recovery, helping to maintain energy levels throughout the day.

3. Listen to Your Body:

- Paying attention to the body's signals and pacing oneself based on how they feel is essential for effective fatigue management. Individuals should prioritize activities that feel manageable and adjust their pace or intensity as needed to prevent fatigue from escalating.

4. Set Realistic Expectations:

- Setting realistic expectations for what can be accomplished in a given timeframe helps prevent disappointment and frustration. Individuals should prioritize essential tasks and accept that some activities may need to be deferred or delegated to conserve energy.

5. Practice Self-Compassion:

- Practicing self-compassion and self-acceptance is crucial for coping with CRF. Individuals should be kind to themselves and acknowledge their limitations without judgment or self-criticism. Accepting help from others and seeking support when needed is a sign of strength, not weakness.

Understanding Goal Setting:

Goal setting involves identifying specific, measurable, achievable, relevant, and time-bound (SMART) objectives to work towards, providing individuals with a sense of purpose, direction, and motivation. Goals serve as benchmarks for progress and accomplishments, helping individuals stay focused and accountable for their actions. Setting goals empowers individuals to take proactive steps towards managing their fatigue and achieving their desired outcomes.

Principles of Goal Setting:

1. Be Specific and Measurable:

   - Setting specific and measurable goals provides clarity and direction, enabling individuals to track their progress and celebrate their achievements. Goals should be concrete, tangible, and achievable within a defined timeframe to maintain motivation and momentum.

2. Set Realistic and Achievable Goals:

   - Setting realistic and achievable goals ensures that individuals can attain success and build confidence in their abilities. Goals should stretch individuals beyond their comfort zone while remaining within the realm of possibility, fostering a sense of accomplishment and self-efficacy.

3. Align Goals with Values and Priorities:

   - Aligning goals with personal values and

priorities ensures that individuals are working towards outcomes that are meaningful and relevant to them. Goals should reflect individuals' aspirations, interests, and needs, providing intrinsic motivation and satisfaction.

4. Break Goals into Actionable Steps:

- Breaking goals into actionable steps helps individuals overcome barriers and obstacles, making progress more manageable and attainable. Each step should be clear, achievable, and linked to the overarching goal, facilitating a sense of progress and accomplishment.

5. Track Progress and Adjust as Needed:

- Tracking progress towards goals and adjusting strategies as needed ensures that individuals stay on course and make continuous improvements. Regular review and reflection enable individuals to celebrate successes, learn from setbacks, and refine their approach to goal achievement.

Benefits of Pacing Activities and Goal Setting:

1. Conserved Energy and Reduced Fatigue:

- Pacing activities and goal setting help individuals conserve energy, prevent overexertion, and reduce fatigue-related distress. By breaking tasks into manageable segments and setting realistic goals, individuals can maintain a balance between activity and rest, optimizing their energy levels and functional capacity.

2. Increased Sense of Control and Empowerment:

- Pacing activities and goal setting empower individuals to take an active role in managing their fatigue and achieving their desired outcomes. By setting priorities, establishing routines, and monitoring progress, individuals gain a sense of control over their lives and a greater sense of self-efficacy.

3. Enhanced Quality of Life and Well-Being:

- Pacing activities and goal setting improve quality of life and well-being by promoting engagement in meaningful activities, fostering a sense of accomplishment and satisfaction, and reducing the impact of fatigue on daily functioning. By pacing themselves and setting achievable goals, individuals can maintain their independence, autonomy, and overall well-being.

Considerations for Implementation:

1. Individualization:

- Pacing activities and goal setting should be tailored to the individual needs, preferences, and circumstances of each cancer patient and survivor. Healthcare providers should collaborate with patients to identify strategies that are feasible, acceptable, and effective for managing CRF.

2. Education and Support:

- Education and support are essential for empowering individuals to implement pacing activities and goal setting effectively. Healthcare providers should provide guidance on pacing techniques, SMART goal setting, and self-monitoring, as well as offer encouragement, reassurance, and practical tips for success.

3. Multidisciplinary Collaboration:

-     Multidisciplinary collaboration among healthcare providers, including physicians, nurses, occupational therapists, physical therapists, and psychologists, is essential for comprehensive fatigue management. Collaborative care ensures that patients receive integrated, holistic support that addresses their unique needs and circumstances.

4. Patient Engagement and Adherence:

- Patient engagement and adherence are critical for the success of pacing activities and goal setting interventions. Healthcare providers should involve patients in decision-making, provide clear instructions and expectations, and offer ongoing support and encouragement to promote adherence and motivation.

Relaxation and Mindfulness Practices

In the face of challenges posed by CRF, relaxation and mindfulness practices offer powerful tools for managing CRF and enhancing overall quality of life.

Understanding Relaxation and Mindfulness:

Relaxation involves intentionally engaging in activities or techniques that promote a state of calmness and relaxation, reducing stress and tension in the body and mind. Mindfulness, on the other hand, is the practice of paying deliberate, non-judgmental attention to the present moment, cultivating awareness, acceptance, and inner peace. Together, relaxation and mindfulness form a synergistic approach to coping with CRF, helping individuals manage symptoms, build resilience, and improve overall well-being.

Principles of Relaxation and Mindfulness:

1. Awareness and Presence:

 - Both relaxation and mindfulness practices emphasize the importance of awareness and presence, encouraging individuals to tune into their thoughts, feelings, and bodily sensations without judgment or attachment. By cultivating present-moment awareness, individuals can reduce rumination, worry, and anxiety, promoting a sense of calmness and clarity.

2. Acceptance and Non-Resistance:

 - Relaxation and mindfulness involve accepting and embracing whatever arises in the present moment, including difficult emotions, physical discomfort, and challenging circumstances. By practicing non-resistance and letting go of the need for control, individuals can reduce suffering and cultivate greater peace and equanimity.

3. Breath Awareness and Regulation:

   - Breath awareness and regulation are central to both relaxation and mindfulness practices, serving as anchors for attention and sources of relaxation and vitality. Deep breathing exercises, such as diaphragmatic breathing and mindful breathing, help activate the body's relaxation response, reduce stress hormones, and promote relaxation and well-being.

4. Body Scan and Progressive Muscle Relaxation:

   - Body scan and progressive muscle relaxation are relaxation techniques that involve systematically tensing and relaxing muscle groups throughout the body, promoting physical and mental relaxation. These practices help release tension, reduce muscle stiffness, and enhance overall relaxation and well-being.

5. Mindful Movement and Yoga:

   - Mindful movement practices, such as yoga, tai chi, and qigong, integrate movement with breath awareness and mindfulness, promoting relaxation, flexibility, and inner peace. These practices help individuals connect mind and body, improve physical functioning, and reduce stress and fatigue.

Benefits of Relaxation and Mindfulness:

1. Stress Reduction and Relaxation:

- Relaxation and mindfulness practices help reduce stress, tension, and anxiety, promoting a sense of relaxation and well-being. By activating the body's relaxation response, these practices lower blood pressure, heart rate, and cortisol levels, fostering a state of calmness and tranquility.

2. Pain Management and Symptom Relief:

- Relaxation and mindfulness techniques have been shown to alleviate pain, discomfort, and other physical symptoms associated with cancer and its treatments. By promoting relaxation, reducing muscle tension, and enhancing pain tolerance, these practices provide natural, non-pharmacological approaches to pain management and symptom relief.

3. Improved Sleep Quality:

- Relaxation and mindfulness practices support restful sleep by calming the mind, relaxing the body, and promoting a sense of ease and relaxation. By incorporating relaxation techniques into bedtime routines, individuals can improve sleep quality, enhance sleep duration, and reduce insomnia and sleep disturbances.

4. Enhanced Emotional Well-Being:

- Relaxation and mindfulness practices foster emotional well-being by promoting self-awareness, acceptance, and emotional regulation. By cultivating mindfulness, individuals can develop greater resilience, cope more effectively with difficult emotions, and foster a greater sense of peace and equanimity.

5. Cognitive Functioning and Mental Clarity:

- Relaxation and mindfulness practices improve cognitive functioning and mental clarity by reducing mental fatigue, enhancing focus and attention, and promoting cognitive flexibility. By training the mind to be present and attentive, these practices support mental acuity, memory, and executive functioning.

Considerations for Implementation:

1. Consistency and Persistence:

- Consistency and persistence are key to deriving maximum benefit from relaxation and mindfulness practices. Individuals should make a commitment to regular practice, incorporating these techniques into their daily routines and making adjustments as needed to maintain motivation and engagement.

2. Integration into Daily Life:

- Relaxation and mindfulness practices can be integrated into various aspects of daily life, including morning routines, work breaks, mealtimes, and bedtime rituals. By incorporating these practices into everyday activities, individuals can create a sense of continuity and presence throughout the day.

3. Adaptation and Flexibility:

- Relaxation and mindfulness practices can

be adapted and customized to suit individual preferences, needs, and circumstances. Individuals should experiment with different techniques and approaches, exploring what resonates with them and adjusting their practice as needed to optimize effectiveness and enjoyment.

4. Support and Community:

- Support and community play an important role in sustaining motivation and engagement with relaxation and mindfulness practices. Individuals should seek out opportunities for connection and support, such as joining mindfulness groups, attending classes or workshops, and participating in online communities.

CHAPTER 6: SUPPORT SYSTEMS FOR COPING WITH CANCER-RELATED FATIGUE

Support systems play a crucial role in helping individuals cope with cancer-related fatigue (CRF). These systems can include family members, friends, support groups, healthcare professionals, and community resources. Family and friends provide emotional support, practical assistance, and encouragement, helping individuals navigate the challenges of CRF with greater resilience. Support groups offer opportunities for connection, validation, and shared experiences, reducing feelings of isolation and fostering a sense of belonging. Healthcare professionals provide guidance, education, and personalized interventions to manage CRF effectively, empowering individuals to take an active role in their care. Community resources, such as cancer centers, wellness programs, and online forums, offer additional support and information, complementing formal medical treatments and enhancing overall well-being. By cultivating strong support systems, individuals with CRF can feel empowered, understood, and equipped to face the challenges of cancer treatment and recovery with greater confidence and resilience.

Role of Support Groups and Peer Support

Support groups and peer support offer invaluable resources for individuals navigating the complexities of CRF.

Understanding Support Groups and Peer Support:

Support groups are structured gatherings of individuals who share common experiences, challenges, or goals related to cancer and its treatments. Peer support involves one-on-one interactions between individuals with similar experiences, providing empathy, understanding, and practical advice. Both support groups and peer support offer opportunities for emotional expression, validation, information sharing, and social connection, fostering a sense of belonging and camaraderie among participants.

Benefits of Support Groups and Peer Support:

1. Emotional Support:
   - Support groups and peer support provide a safe and non-judgmental space for individuals to express their feelings, fears, and frustrations related to CRF. Sharing experiences with others who understand can reduce feelings of isolation, shame, and distress, promoting emotional healing and resilience.

2. Practical Advice and Coping Strategies:

- Support groups and peer support offer opportunities for individuals to exchange practical advice, tips, and coping strategies for managing CRF. Participants can learn from each other's experiences, gather information about available resources, and explore alternative approaches to symptom management.

3. Sense of Belonging and Community:

- Participation in support groups and peer support fosters a sense of belonging and community among individuals affected by CRF. Knowing that they are not alone in their experiences can provide comfort, validation, and hope, reducing feelings of alienation and despair.

4. Information Sharing and Education:

- Support groups and peer support serve as valuable sources of information and education about CRF and its management. Participants can learn about the latest research, treatments, and supportive care interventions, empowering them to make informed decisions about their health and well-being.

5. Empowerment and Advocacy:

- Support groups and peer support empower individuals to become active participants in their care and advocates for themselves and others affected by CRF. By sharing their stories, raising awareness, and advocating for better support and resources, participants can effect positive change in their communities and healthcare systems.

Structure and Implementation of Support Groups and Peer Support:

1. Facilitated Discussions:
   - Support groups are typically facilitated by trained professionals, such as social workers, psychologists, or oncology nurses, who guide discussions, ensure a supportive environment, and provide resources and information as needed. Peer support may be facilitated by volunteers or trained peer mentors who have firsthand experience with CRF.

2. Structured Meetings:
   - Support groups may meet regularly, either in person or virtually, to discuss specific topics, share experiences, and engage in supportive activities. Meetings may include structured discussions, guest speakers, educational presentations, or experiential exercises designed to promote healing and empowerment.

3. Confidentiality and Respect:
   - Support groups and peer support programs prioritize confidentiality, respect, and privacy, creating a safe space for participants to share their thoughts and feelings without fear of judgment or reprisal. Ground rules for participation, including guidelines for confidentiality and respectful communication, are established and enforced to

maintain a supportive atmosphere.

4. Accessibility and Inclusivity:

- Support groups and peer support programs strive to be accessible and inclusive to individuals from diverse backgrounds, cultures, and experiences. Efforts are made to accommodate participants' needs and preferences, including providing language interpretation, wheelchair accessibility, and online options for participation.

Considerations for Participation:

1. Choosing the Right Group:

- Individuals should choose support groups or peer support programs that align with their needs, preferences, and goals. Factors to consider include the format, location, membership, and focus of the group, as well as the qualifications and expertise of the facilitators or mentors.

2. Setting Boundaries:

- Participants should set boundaries and manage their expectations regarding their involvement in support groups or peer support programs. It is important to balance participation with self-care and to respect the privacy and boundaries of others within the group.

3. Managing Emotional Triggers:

- Support group participants may encounter emotional triggers or distressing content during discussions. It is essential to have coping strategies in place to manage emotional reactions, such as deep breathing, mindfulness techniques, or seeking support from a trusted friend or mental health professional.

4. Seeking Professional Support:
   - While support groups and peer support can be valuable sources of support, they are not a substitute for professional medical or psychological care. Individuals experiencing significant distress or mental health concerns should seek support from a qualified healthcare provider or mental health professional.

Communicating with Healthcare Providers and Loved Ones

Effective communication is a cornerstone of coping with cancer-related fatigue (CRF), both with healthcare providers and loved ones. Open, honest, and compassionate dialogue can facilitate understanding, support, and shared decision-making, empowering individuals to navigate the challenges of CRF with greater resilience and confidence.

Communication with Healthcare Providers:

1. Openness and Transparency:
   - Effective communication with healthcare providers begins with openness and transparency.

Individuals should feel comfortable sharing their concerns, symptoms, and experiences related to CRF, providing valuable insights that guide treatment decisions and interventions.

2. Active Participation:

- Individuals should actively participate in discussions with their healthcare providers, asking questions, seeking clarification, and expressing their preferences and goals for managing CRF. Collaborative decision-making promotes a sense of ownership and empowerment, enhancing engagement and adherence to treatment plans.

3. Symptom Management:

- Clear communication with healthcare providers is essential for identifying and addressing symptoms of CRF effectively. Individuals should report changes in fatigue levels, functional abilities, and quality of life, enabling healthcare providers to tailor interventions and support strategies to their unique needs and circumstances.

4. Treatment Preferences:

- Individuals should communicate their treatment preferences and priorities with their healthcare providers, including their willingness to try different approaches, their concerns about potential side effects, and their goals for maintaining quality of life. Shared decision-making ensures that treatment plans align with individuals' values and preferences, fostering a sense of partnership and trust.

5. Follow-Up and Feedback:

- Regular follow-up and feedback are essential for ongoing communication with healthcare providers. Individuals should provide feedback about the effectiveness of interventions, share any concerns or challenges they encounter, and collaborate with their providers to adjust treatment plans as needed to optimize outcomes and well-being.

Communication with Loved Ones:

1. Open Dialogue:

- Open dialogue with loved ones is essential for navigating the emotional and practical challenges of CRF. Individuals should feel comfortable discussing their experiences, fears, and needs with their loved ones, fostering mutual understanding, empathy, and support.

2. Educational Support:

- Loved ones can provide valuable educational support by learning about CRF and its impact on individuals' lives. By gaining knowledge and awareness, loved ones can offer informed support, validate individuals' experiences, and provide practical assistance as needed.

3. Emotional Support:

- Emotional support from loved ones is a vital source of comfort and strength for individuals coping with CRF. Listening with empathy, offering words of encouragement, and expressing love and affection can help alleviate feelings of isolation, fear, and distress, promoting emotional healing and resilience.

4. Practical Assistance:

- Practical assistance from loved ones can help alleviate the burden of CRF and facilitate daily functioning and well-being. From helping with household chores and transportation to providing emotional support and companionship, loved ones play a crucial role in supporting individuals' physical, emotional, and social needs.

5. Boundaries and Self-Care:

- While support from loved ones is invaluable, it is essential for individuals to set boundaries and prioritize self-care to avoid caregiver burnout and maintain balance in their relationships. Open communication about needs, expectations, and limitations fosters mutual respect and understanding, enhancing the quality of relationships and support.

Benefits of Effective Communication:

1. Improved Symptom Management:

- Effective communication with healthcare providers facilitates the identification and management of symptoms of CRF, leading to better outcomes and quality of life for individuals affected by this condition.

2. Enhanced Emotional Support:

- Open dialogue with loved ones fosters emotional support and connection, reducing feelings of isolation, anxiety, and depression, and promoting emotional well-being and resilience.

3. Shared Decision-Making:

- Collaborative communication with healthcare providers enables shared decision-making and patient-centered care, ensuring that treatment plans align with individuals' values, preferences, and goals.

4. Empowerment and Advocacy:

- Effective communication empowers individuals to advocate for themselves, assert their needs, and actively participate in their care, promoting a sense of empowerment, autonomy, and self-efficacy.

5. Strengthened Relationships:

- Open, honest, and compassionate communication fosters trust, understanding, and intimacy in relationships with healthcare providers and loved ones, strengthening social support networks and enhancing overall well-being.

Strategies for Effective Communication:

1. Active Listening:

- Practice active listening by giving your full attention, maintaining eye contact, and providing verbal and nonverbal cues that you are engaged and interested in what the other person is saying.

2. Clarification and Summarization:

- Clarify understanding by asking questions, seeking clarification, and summarizing key points to ensure that both parties are on the same page and have a shared understanding of the conversation.

3. Empathy and Validation:

- Express empathy and validation by acknowledging the other person's feelings, experiences, and perspectives, even if you may not fully understand or agree with them. Validate their emotions and experiences as valid and worthy of consideration.

4. Use of "I" Statements:

- Use "I" statements to express your thoughts, feelings, and needs in a non-confrontational and assertive manner, focusing on your own experiences rather than blaming or accusing the other person.

5. Problem-Solving and Collaboration:

- Approach communication as a collaborative problem-solving process, working together with the other person to identify solutions, address concerns, and achieve mutually satisfactory outcomes.

Available Resources for Coping with Fatigue

Coping with fatigue, especially in the context of

cancer-related fatigue (CRF), requires a multifaceted approach that often involves tapping into various resources and support systems. Here are several resources available for individuals coping with fatigue:

1. Healthcare Providers and Treatment Teams:

Healthcare providers, including oncologists, nurses, and other members of the treatment team, serve as primary resources for managing fatigue. They can offer medical interventions, such as medications or adjustments to treatment regimens, to address underlying causes of fatigue. Additionally, they provide guidance on lifestyle modifications, symptom management techniques, and referrals to supportive care services.

2. Support Groups and Peer Support Programs:

Support groups and peer support programs provide valuable emotional and practical support for individuals experiencing fatigue. These groups offer a safe space for sharing experiences, expressing concerns, and accessing peer-driven insights and coping strategies. Whether in-person or online, support groups foster a sense of community and understanding among participants, reducing feelings of isolation and providing validation for individuals' experiences.

3. Educational Resources and Informational Materials:

Educational resources and informational

materials, such as pamphlets, websites, and online forums, offer valuable insights and practical tips for managing fatigue. These resources may cover topics ranging from understanding the underlying causes of fatigue to implementing lifestyle modifications and self-care strategies. By educating themselves about fatigue and its management, individuals can empower themselves to make informed decisions and take proactive steps towards improving their well-being.

4. Psychosocial Support Services:

Psychosocial support services, including counseling, psychotherapy, and mindfulness-based interventions, address the emotional and psychological aspects of fatigue. Mental health professionals can help individuals navigate the emotional impact of fatigue, cope with stress and anxiety, and develop resilience and coping skills. These services offer a holistic approach to fatigue management, addressing the interconnectedness of physical, emotional, and social well-being.

5. Exercise and Rehabilitation Programs:

Exercise and rehabilitation programs, tailored to individuals' needs and abilities, can help alleviate fatigue and improve overall functioning and quality of life. These programs may include aerobic exercise, strength training, yoga, and tai chi, which have been shown to reduce fatigue, increase energy levels, and enhance physical and emotional well-being. Additionally, physical therapists and exercise specialists can provide guidance on safe and effective exercise routines for individuals affected by fatigue.

6. Nutritional Support and Dietary Counseling:

Nutritional support and dietary counseling play a crucial role in managing fatigue by addressing nutritional deficiencies, promoting healthy eating habits, and optimizing energy levels. Registered dietitians can assess individuals' nutritional needs, provide personalized dietary recommendations, and offer practical strategies for maintaining a balanced diet despite fatigue-related challenges. By fueling their bodies with nourishing foods, individuals can support their overall health and vitality.

7. Complementary and Integrative Therapies:

Complementary and integrative therapies, such as acupuncture, massage therapy, and herbal supplements, offer alternative approaches to managing fatigue and promoting relaxation and well-being. While research on the efficacy of these therapies for fatigue is ongoing, many individuals find relief from symptoms and enjoy improved quality of life through their use. It's essential to consult with healthcare providers before incorporating complementary therapies into one's treatment plan to ensure safety and compatibility with existing treatments.

8. Caregiver and Family Support Programs:

Caregiver and family support programs provide resources and assistance for caregivers who are supporting individuals experiencing fatigue. These programs offer education, respite care, and emotional support to help caregivers navigate the challenges of caregiving while maintaining their own well-being. By addressing the needs of caregivers, these programs contribute to a supportive and nurturing environment for individuals affected by fatigue.

CHAPTER 7: NAVIGATING WORK AND DAILY LIFE WITH CANCER-RELATED FATIGUE

Navigating work and daily life while managing cancer-related fatigue (CRF) requires a delicate balance of self-care, communication, and adaptation. Individuals affected by CRF often find it helpful to prioritize tasks, delegate responsibilities when possible, and establish realistic expectations for their energy levels and abilities. Open communication with employers, coworkers, and loved ones about the challenges of CRF can facilitate understanding and support, enabling individuals to access accommodations, modify work schedules, or seek assistance as needed. Additionally, incorporating rest breaks, practicing energy conservation techniques, and implementing stress-reduction strategies throughout the day can help individuals manage fatigue and maintain productivity and well-being. By embracing self-compassion, flexibility, and proactive self-care, individuals can navigate the demands of work and daily life with greater resilience and empowerment despite the challenges posed by CRF.

Managing Fatigue in the Workplace

Managing fatigue in the workplace, particularly in the context of cancer-related fatigue (CRF), is essential for maintaining productivity, well-being, and job satisfaction. CRF can significantly impact individuals' ability to perform tasks, concentrate, and engage in work-related activities, presenting unique challenges for both employees and employers.

Understanding Cancer-Related Fatigue in the Workplace:

Cancer-related fatigue (CRF) is a pervasive and distressing symptom experienced by many cancer patients and survivors, affecting physical, emotional, and cognitive functioning. In the workplace, CRF can manifest as reduced energy levels, difficulty concentrating, impaired memory, and increased sensitivity to environmental stimuli. These symptoms can interfere with job performance, productivity, and overall well-being, posing challenges for individuals striving to maintain employment and meet job demands.

Strategies for Managing Fatigue in the Workplace:

1. Open Communication:
   - Open communication between employees and employers is essential for addressing the challenges of CRF in the workplace. Individuals affected by CRF should feel comfortable discussing their symptoms, needs, and limitations with their supervisors, HR

departments, and colleagues, enabling them to access support and accommodations as needed.

2. Flexible Work Arrangements:

-   Flexible work arrangements, such as telecommuting, flexible hours, and modified schedules, can help individuals manage fatigue and balance work responsibilities with rest and self-care. Employers can work with employees to explore alternative work arrangements that accommodate their energy levels and optimize productivity and well-being.

3. Accommodations and Workplace Adjustments:

-   Employers can provide accommodations and workplace adjustments to support individuals affected by CRF in performing their job duties effectively. This may include ergonomic modifications, assistive devices, noise reduction measures, and access to quiet spaces for rest breaks. By addressing environmental barriers and reducing physical and cognitive demands, employers can create a supportive and inclusive work environment for individuals with CRF.

4. Job Redesign and Task Delegation:

-   Job redesign and task delegation can help individuals with CRF manage their workload more effectively by reallocating responsibilities and streamlining tasks. Employers can work with employees to identify essential job functions, prioritize tasks, and delegate non-essential or physically demanding duties to other team members. By redistributing workload and adjusting job responsibilities, employers can help individuals with CRF maintain productivity and job satisfaction.

5. Education and Training:

   - Education and training programs can raise awareness about CRF in the workplace and provide employees and employers with knowledge and skills for managing fatigue effectively. Employers can offer training sessions on fatigue management techniques, stress reduction strategies, and ergonomics principles, empowering employees to take proactive steps towards maintaining their health and well-being at work.

6. Self-Care Practices:

   - Self-care practices are essential for managing fatigue in the workplace and promoting overall well-being. Individuals with CRF can incorporate self-care activities into their daily routine, such as taking regular breaks, practicing relaxation techniques, staying hydrated, and engaging in gentle exercise. By prioritizing self-care and listening to their bodies' signals, individuals can conserve energy, reduce stress, and enhance resilience in the face of CRF.

7. Social Support Networks:

   - Social support networks, including colleagues, supervisors, and employee assistance programs, offer valuable emotional and practical support for individuals with CRF in the workplace. Colleagues can provide encouragement, understanding, and assistance with tasks, while supervisors and HR departments can facilitate access to resources and accommodations. Employee assistance programs may offer counseling, coaching, and referrals to additional support services to help employees cope with the challenges of CRF.

Organizational Policies and Best Practices:

1. Fatigue Management Policies:
-    Organizations can implement fatigue management policies and best practices to support employees affected by CRF. These policies may include guidelines for requesting accommodations, procedures for documenting fatigue-related concerns, and resources for accessing support services. By formalizing procedures and promoting awareness, organizations can create a supportive and inclusive work environment for individuals with CRF.

2. Workplace Wellness Programs:
- Workplace wellness programs can promote employee health and well-being by offering resources, incentives, and activities focused on fatigue management and stress reduction. These programs may include educational workshops, fitness classes, mindfulness sessions, and access to wellness resources and tools. By investing

in employee wellness, organizations can foster a culture of health and productivity, benefiting both employees and the organization as a whole.

3. Employee Assistance Programs (EAPs):
   - Employee assistance programs (EAPs) provide confidential counseling, support, and resources for employees facing personal or work-related challenges, including fatigue-related concerns. EAPs offer access to licensed counselors, mental health professionals, and other support services to help employees cope with the physical, emotional, and practical aspects of CRF. By providing confidential and accessible support, EAPs can empower employees to address fatigue-related concerns proactively and effectively.

Balancing Responsibilities and Coping with Fatigue

Balancing responsibilities while coping with fatigue is a common challenge faced by many individuals, especially those dealing with conditions like cancer-related fatigue (CRF). Juggling work, family obligations, social commitments, and self-care needs can feel overwhelming when energy levels are depleted. However, by implementing effective strategies and prioritizing self-care, individuals can navigate life's demands while managing fatigue more effectively.

Understanding the Impact of Fatigue on Daily Life:

Fatigue, whether related to medical conditions, stress, or lifestyle factors, can significantly impact daily functioning and quality of life. Individuals experiencing fatigue may struggle with concentration, motivation, physical stamina, and emotional resilience, making it challenging to fulfill responsibilities and engage in activities they enjoy. Fatigue can affect performance at work, strain relationships, and limit participation in social and recreational pursuits, leading to feelings of frustration, guilt, and isolation.

Strategies for Balancing Responsibilities and Coping with Fatigue:

1. Prioritize Self-Care:
   - Prioritizing self-care is essential for managing fatigue and maintaining overall well-being. Individuals should make time for rest, relaxation, and activities that rejuvenate their mind, body, and spirit. This may include practicing mindfulness, engaging in hobbies, getting quality sleep, and nourishing the body with healthy food and hydration.

2. Set Realistic Expectations:
   - Setting realistic expectations for oneself is crucial when managing fatigue. Individuals should acknowledge their limitations and adjust their goals and expectations accordingly. Breaking tasks into smaller, manageable steps and celebrating progress, no matter how small, can help individuals feel

accomplished and motivated despite fatigue-related challenges.

3. Delegate Tasks and Seek Support:

- Delegating tasks and seeking support from others can lighten the load and reduce stress for individuals coping with fatigue. Whether at work or home, individuals can enlist the help of colleagues, family members, or friends to share responsibilities and provide assistance as needed. Effective communication and clear delegation of tasks can ensure that everyone understands their role and contributes to shared goals.

4. Practice Time Management:

- Effective time management is key to balancing responsibilities and conserving energy. Individuals can use tools such as calendars, planners, and to-do lists to prioritize tasks, allocate time efficiently, and avoid overcommitting themselves. Setting boundaries, saying no to non-essential commitments, and scheduling regular breaks can help individuals manage their energy levels and prevent burnout.

5. Employ Energy Conservation Techniques:

- Energy conservation techniques involve pacing activities, prioritizing tasks, and minimizing unnecessary exertion to preserve energy throughout the day. Individuals can identify their peak energy periods and schedule demanding tasks during these times, while reserving low-energy periods for rest or less demanding activities. Taking short breaks, practicing relaxation techniques, and avoiding multitasking can also help conserve energy and prevent fatigue accumulation.

6. Seek Accommodations and Flexibility:

- Individuals experiencing fatigue may benefit from accommodations and flexibility in their work or academic environments. This may include flexible work hours, telecommuting options, ergonomic adjustments, or modified workloads to accommodate fluctuating energy levels and optimize productivity. Open communication with supervisors, educators, or healthcare providers can facilitate the implementation of accommodations tailored to individuals' needs.

7. Engage in Stress Reduction Activities:

- Stress reduction activities, such as mindfulness meditation, deep breathing exercises, and yoga, can help individuals manage fatigue and promote relaxation and resilience. These practices reduce the physiological and psychological effects of stress, improve coping skills, and enhance overall well-being. Incorporating stress reduction activities into daily routines can foster a sense of calmness and balance amidst life's demands.

8. Maintain Social Connections:

- Maintaining social connections is essential for emotional support and resilience when coping with fatigue. Individuals should prioritize spending time with supportive friends, family members, or peers who understand their challenges and provide encouragement and companionship. Connecting with others through social activities, support groups, or online communities can help combat feelings of isolation and foster a sense of belonging and connection.

Emotional Impact on Daily Life and Relationships

The emotional impact of fatigue on daily life and relationships can be profound, affecting individuals' mood, well-being, and interpersonal dynamics. Whether stemming from medical conditions, stress, or lifestyle factors, fatigue can influence how individuals perceive themselves, interact with others, and navigate life's challenges.

Understanding the Emotional Effects of Fatigue:

Fatigue can elicit a range of emotional responses, including frustration, irritability, sadness, anxiety, and guilt. Individuals experiencing fatigue may feel frustrated by their limited energy levels, resentful of the tasks they are unable to accomplish, and anxious about their ability to meet responsibilities. Moreover, fatigue can erode self-esteem and self-efficacy, leading individuals to question their competence, worthiness, and identity.

In addition to its individual effects, fatigue can

strain relationships and interpersonal dynamics. Partners, family members, friends, and colleagues may struggle to understand the impact of fatigue on individuals' lives, leading to misunderstandings, conflicts, and feelings of resentment or isolation. Moreover, individuals affected by fatigue may withdraw from social interactions, reduce participation in activities, and experience feelings of loneliness and disconnection from others.

Coping Strategies for Managing Emotional Impact:

1. Self-Compassion and Acceptance:

   - Practicing self-compassion and acceptance is crucial when coping with the emotional impact of fatigue. Individuals should acknowledge their limitations, validate their experiences, and offer themselves kindness and understanding. Cultivating self-compassion fosters resilience and self-worth, allowing individuals to navigate challenges with greater ease and grace.

2. Emotional Regulation Techniques:

   - Learning and practicing emotional regulation techniques can help individuals manage difficult emotions associated with fatigue. Techniques such as deep breathing, mindfulness meditation, and progressive muscle relaxation can promote relaxation, reduce stress, and enhance emotional well-being. By cultivating awareness of their emotions and developing coping skills, individuals can respond to fatigue-related challenges with greater equanimity and resilience.

3. Effective Communication:

- Effective communication is essential for navigating the emotional impact of fatigue on relationships. Individuals should openly communicate with their loved ones about their experiences, needs, and limitations, fostering understanding, empathy, and support. Honest and compassionate dialogue enables individuals to express their feelings, set boundaries, and seek assistance when needed, strengthening interpersonal connections and promoting mutual respect and cooperation.

4. Setting Realistic Expectations:

- Setting realistic expectations for oneself and others is key to managing the emotional impact of fatigue. Individuals should recognize that they may not be able to accomplish as much as they would like when experiencing fatigue and adjust their expectations accordingly. By setting achievable goals, prioritizing self-care, and celebrating small victories, individuals can cultivate a sense of accomplishment and fulfillment amidst fatigue-related challenges.

5. Seeking Support:

- Seeking support from others can provide validation, encouragement, and perspective when coping with the emotional impact of fatigue. Whether from friends, family members, support groups, or mental health professionals, support networks offer invaluable resources and emotional support. Sharing experiences, receiving validation, and accessing practical assistance can help individuals feel less alone and more empowered to navigate fatigue-related challenges.

6. Engaging in Self-Care Practices:

- Engaging in self-care practices is essential for maintaining emotional well-being when coping with fatigue. Individuals should prioritize activities that nourish their mind, body, and spirit, such as getting adequate rest, eating nutritious foods, exercising regularly, and engaging in activities they enjoy. By investing in their self-care, individuals can replenish their energy reserves, reduce stress, and enhance resilience in the face of fatigue-related challenges.

Implications for Personal and Interpersonal Growth:

The emotional impact of fatigue on daily life and relationships presents opportunities for personal and interpersonal growth. Individuals affected by fatigue can develop greater self-awareness, emotional intelligence, and resilience as they navigate challenges, cultivate self-compassion, and seek support from others. Moreover, relationships can deepen and strengthen as individuals communicate openly, express vulnerability, and offer empathy and support to one another. By embracing the lessons learned from navigating the emotional impact of fatigue, individuals can foster personal growth, strengthen relationships, and cultivate a greater sense of well-being and fulfillment in their lives.

CHAPTER 8: CANCER SURVIVORSHIP AND LONG-TERM MANAGEMENT OF FATIGUE

Cancer survivorship brings unique challenges, including the long-term management of fatigue. Even after completing treatment, many survivors continue to experience fatigue, impacting their daily life and quality of life. Survivorship care plans often include strategies for managing fatigue, such as regular physical activity, adequate sleep, balanced nutrition, and stress reduction techniques. Additionally, survivors may benefit from support groups, counseling, and healthcare provider follow-up to address ongoing fatigue and related concerns. By prioritizing self-care and accessing appropriate support, cancer survivors can navigate the long-term management of fatigue and optimize their well-being as they transition into life after cancer treatment.

Challenges of Fatigue During and After Treatment

The multifaceted challenges of fatigue during and after cancer treatment, including its physical, emotional, and practical impacts may be overwhelming. We will now discuss strategies for managing fatigue effectively to enhance quality of life and promote overall well-being during and after cancer treatment.

Understanding the Challenges of Fatigue During Treatment:

During cancer treatment, individuals may experience fatigue as a result of various factors, including the effects of chemotherapy, radiation therapy, surgery, and other treatment modalities. Cancer-related fatigue (CRF) is often described as profound tiredness that does not improve with rest and can significantly impact daily functioning and quality of life. The physical toll of treatment, combined with emotional distress, sleep disturbances, and changes in routine, can exacerbate fatigue and make it challenging for individuals to cope effectively.

Furthermore, the unpredictability and variability of fatigue can complicate treatment planning and decision-making, as individuals may struggle to anticipate and manage their energy levels amidst the demands of treatment. Fatigue can also interfere with adherence to treatment regimens, leading to delays, dose reductions, or discontinuation of therapy, which may compromise treatment outcomes and prognosis.

Challenges of Fatigue in Survivorship:

Even after completing cancer treatment, many survivors continue to experience fatigue, impacting their daily life and quality of life. Fatigue during survivorship may be influenced by various factors, including the lingering effects of treatment, ongoing side effects, physical deconditioning, psychological distress, and comorbidities. Additionally, survivors may face challenges such as returning to work, resuming social activities, and adjusting to changes in roles and responsibilities, which can exacerbate fatigue and impair functioning.

Moreover, the emotional toll of cancer survivorship, including fear of recurrence, anxiety, depression, and existential concerns, can contribute to fatigue and exacerbate its impact on daily life. Survivors may struggle to find a sense of normalcy and regain a sense of control over their lives, leading to feelings of frustration, isolation, and hopelessness.

Strategies for Managing Fatigue During and After Treatment:

1. Physical Activity and Exercise:
   - Regular physical activity and exercise can help alleviate fatigue, improve energy levels, and enhance overall well-being during and after cancer treatment. Individuals should aim for a combination of aerobic exercise, strength training, and flexibility exercises tailored to their abilities and preferences. Gradual progression and guidance from healthcare providers or exercise specialists can help individuals safely incorporate exercise into

their routine and optimize its benefits for fatigue management.

2. Sleep Hygiene:

- Prioritizing sleep hygiene is essential for managing fatigue and promoting restorative sleep during and after cancer treatment. Individuals should establish a consistent sleep schedule, create a relaxing bedtime routine, and optimize their sleep environment for comfort and relaxation. Avoiding stimulants such as caffeine and electronics before bedtime, practicing relaxation techniques, and seeking treatment for sleep disturbances can help improve sleep quality and reduce fatigue.

3. Nutrition and Hydration:

- Balanced nutrition and hydration are crucial for supporting energy levels and overall health during cancer treatment and survivorship. Individuals should aim for a well-rounded diet rich in fruits, vegetables, lean proteins, whole grains, and healthy fats, while staying hydrated with plenty of water. Consulting with a registered dietitian can provide personalized guidance on nutrition and hydration strategies to support energy levels and manage fatigue effectively.

4. Stress Reduction Techniques:

- Stress reduction techniques, such as mindfulness meditation, deep breathing exercises, progressive muscle relaxation, and guided imagery, can help individuals cope with the emotional impact of cancer treatment and reduce fatigue. These practices promote relaxation, enhance coping skills, and improve emotional well-being, empowering individuals to navigate the challenges of fatigue with greater resilience and ease.

5. Pacing and Energy Conservation:
- Pacing activities and practicing energy conservation techniques can help individuals manage fatigue by balancing activity and rest throughout the day. Breaking tasks into manageable segments, prioritizing essential activities, and scheduling rest breaks can prevent overexertion and minimize fatigue accumulation. Setting realistic goals, delegating tasks, and seeking assistance when needed can also help individuals conserve energy and optimize their ability to function effectively.

6. Psychosocial Support:
- Psychosocial support, including counseling, support groups, and peer support programs, can provide valuable emotional and practical support for individuals coping with fatigue during and after cancer treatment. Counseling can help individuals address emotional distress, develop coping strategies, and navigate challenges related to fatigue and survivorship. Support groups offer opportunities for connection, validation, and shared experiences with others facing similar challenges, reducing feelings of isolation and fostering a sense of community and belonging.

7. Communication and Advocacy:

- Open communication with healthcare providers, caregivers, and loved ones is essential for addressing the challenges of fatigue during and after cancer treatment. Individuals should feel comfortable expressing their concerns, discussing their symptoms, and seeking support and assistance as needed. Advocating for their needs, preferences, and priorities can help individuals access appropriate resources, accommodations, and support services to manage fatigue effectively and optimize their well-being.

Promoting Long-Term Wellness and Managing Persistent Fatigue

For cancer survivors, promoting long-term wellness and managing persistent fatigue are essential components of post-treatment life. Despite completing treatment, many survivors continue to grapple with fatigue, impacting their overall well-being and quality of life.

Understanding Persistent Fatigue in Survivorship:

Persistent fatigue, commonly experienced by cancer survivors, is characterized by prolonged feelings of tiredness, weakness, and exhaustion that persist beyond treatment completion. This fatigue can stem from various factors, including the physical and psychological effects of cancer and its treatment, sleep disturbances, hormonal changes, and lifestyle factors. Persistent fatigue can significantly impact survivors' ability to function, engage in daily activities, and pursue their goals, posing challenges to their long-term wellness and quality of life.

Strategies for Promoting Long-Term Wellness:

1. Physical Activity and Exercise:
- Engaging in regular physical activity and exercise is crucial for promoting long-term wellness and managing persistent fatigue. Survivors should aim for a combination of aerobic exercise, strength training, and flexibility exercises tailored to their abilities and preferences. Exercise not only improves physical fitness but also enhances mood, energy levels, and overall well-being. Gradual progression and guidance from healthcare providers or exercise specialists can help survivors safely incorporate exercise into their routine and optimize its benefits for fatigue management.

2. Healthy Nutrition and Hydration:
- Adopting a balanced and nutritious diet is essential for supporting energy levels, immune function, and overall health in survivorship. Survivors should prioritize whole foods, including fruits, vegetables, lean proteins, whole grains, and healthy fats, while limiting processed foods, sugary beverages, and excessive alcohol consumption.

Staying hydrated with plenty of water throughout the day is also important for maintaining optimal hydration and combating fatigue.

3. Quality Sleep and Rest:

- Prioritizing quality sleep and restorative rest is essential for managing persistent fatigue and promoting overall well-being. Survivors should establish a consistent sleep schedule, create a relaxing bedtime routine, and optimize their sleep environment for comfort and relaxation. Avoiding stimulants such as caffeine and electronics before bedtime, practicing relaxation techniques, and seeking treatment for sleep disturbances can help improve sleep quality and reduce fatigue.

4. Stress Reduction and Mindfulness:

- Practicing stress reduction techniques and mindfulness meditation can help survivors cope with the emotional impact of cancer survivorship and reduce persistent fatigue. Techniques such as deep breathing exercises, progressive muscle relaxation, and guided imagery promote relaxation, enhance coping skills, and improve emotional well-being. By cultivating mindfulness and awareness of the present moment, survivors can reduce stress, enhance resilience, and manage fatigue more effectively.

5. Pacing and Energy Conservation:

- Pacing activities and practicing energy conservation techniques can help survivors manage persistent fatigue by balancing activity and rest throughout the day. Breaking tasks into manageable segments, prioritizing essential activities, and scheduling rest breaks can prevent overexertion and minimize fatigue accumulation. Setting realistic goals, delegating tasks, and seeking assistance when needed can also help survivors conserve energy and optimize their ability to function effectively.

6. Social Support and Connection:

   - Maintaining social support networks and fostering meaningful connections with others are essential for promoting long-term wellness and managing persistent fatigue. Survivors should seek support from friends, family members, support groups, and mental health professionals who understand their experiences and provide empathy, encouragement, and validation. Connecting with others through social activities, hobbies, and shared interests can reduce feelings of isolation and enhance overall well-being.

7. Regular Healthcare Follow-Up:

   - Regular healthcare follow-up and monitoring are crucial for managing persistent fatigue and addressing any underlying medical or psychological concerns. Survivors should attend scheduled follow-up appointments with their healthcare providers, discuss any ongoing symptoms or concerns related to fatigue, and receive appropriate assessments and interventions as needed. Healthcare providers can offer guidance, support, and referrals to additional resources or specialists to optimize survivors' well-being and quality of life.

Survivorship Care Plans and Follow-Up Care

Survivorship care plans and follow-up strategies play a vital role in ensuring the long-term health and well-being of cancer survivors. As individuals transition from active treatment to survivorship, they face unique challenges and needs that require ongoing support, monitoring, and coordination of care.

Understanding Survivorship Care Plans:

Survivorship care plans are comprehensive documents that outline a roadmap for post-treatment care and support tailored to each survivor's individual needs. These plans typically include a summary of the survivor's cancer diagnosis, treatment history, potential long-term effects or late effects of treatment, recommended follow-up care guidelines, strategies for managing side effects, and resources for support and survivorship programs.

Key Components of Survivorship Care Plans:

1. Treatment Summary:
   - The treatment summary provides an overview of the survivor's cancer diagnosis, including the type and stage of cancer, treatments received

(e.g., surgery, chemotherapy, radiation therapy), and dates of treatment. This summary serves as a reference point for healthcare providers involved in the survivor's ongoing care and facilitates communication and coordination among members of the survivor's healthcare team.

2. Follow-Up Care Guidelines:
-   Follow-up care guidelines outline recommendations for ongoing surveillance, monitoring, and preventive care to detect and manage potential late effects or complications of cancer treatment. These guidelines may include recommendations for regular physical examinations, imaging studies, laboratory tests, and screenings for cancer recurrence, as well as management of comorbidities and health promotion activities.

3. Management of Late Effects:
- Survivorship care plans address the potential long-term effects or late effects of cancer treatment, such as fatigue, pain, cognitive changes, neuropathy, cardiovascular complications, and psychological distress. Strategies for managing late effects may include lifestyle modifications, symptom management techniques, rehabilitative therapies, psychosocial support services, and referrals to specialty providers as needed.

4. Health Promotion and Wellness:
-   Health promotion and wellness

recommendations emphasize the importance of adopting healthy lifestyle behaviors to optimize survivors' overall health and quality of life. These recommendations may include guidance on nutrition, physical activity, smoking cessation, alcohol moderation, stress reduction, sleep hygiene, and adherence to preventive care measures (e.g., vaccinations, screenings).

5. Psychosocial Support Resources:

- Survivorship care plans provide information on psychosocial support resources, survivorship programs, support groups, counseling services, and community-based organizations that offer emotional support, education, and resources for survivors and their families. Access to psychosocial support can help survivors cope with the emotional impact of cancer, reduce distress, and improve overall well-being.

Importance of Follow-Up Care:

Follow-up care is essential for monitoring survivors' health, detecting potential cancer recurrence or late effects of treatment, addressing ongoing medical and psychosocial needs, and promoting overall wellness. Regular follow-up appointments with healthcare providers allow survivors to receive personalized assessments, screenings, interventions, and education tailored to their individual needs and circumstances.

Benefits of Follow-Up Care:

1. Early Detection and Intervention:
   - Regular follow-up care facilitates early detection and intervention for potential cancer recurrence, late effects of treatment, and other health concerns. Timely detection of changes in survivors' health status enables healthcare providers to initiate appropriate diagnostic evaluations, treatments, and supportive interventions to optimize outcomes and quality of life.

2. Monitoring of Treatment Effects:
   - Follow-up care allows healthcare providers to monitor the effects of cancer treatment on survivors' physical, emotional, and psychosocial well-being over time. By tracking survivors' progress and addressing emerging issues or concerns, healthcare providers can tailor interventions and support services to meet survivors' evolving needs and preferences.

3. Coordination of Care:
   - Follow-up care promotes coordination and continuity of care among survivors' healthcare providers, ensuring seamless communication, collaboration, and integration of services. Healthcare providers can share information, coordinate referrals, and collaborate on survivorship care plans to address survivors' comprehensive needs and optimize care delivery.

4. Education and Empowerment:
   - Follow-up care provides opportunities for

survivors to receive education, information, and resources to empower them to actively participate in their own care and self-management. Healthcare providers can offer guidance on managing treatment-related side effects, adopting healthy lifestyle behaviors, accessing support services, and making informed decisions about their health and well-being.

5. Supportive Relationships:

- Follow-up care fosters supportive relationships between survivors and their healthcare providers, creating a safe and trusting environment for open communication, shared decision-making, and mutual respect. Building rapport and trust with healthcare providers encourages survivors to voice their concerns, ask questions, and seek assistance when needed, enhancing their overall experience of care.

CHAPTER 9: FUTURE DIRECTIONS IN CANCER-RELATED FATIGUE RESEARCH AND TREATMENT

Future directions in cancer-related fatigue research and treatment hold promise for improving the quality of life for cancer survivors. Research efforts are focusing on gaining a deeper understanding of the underlying mechanisms of fatigue, including biological, psychological, and social factors, to develop more targeted interventions. Additionally, advancements in technology and personalized medicine offer opportunities to tailor fatigue management strategies to individual needs and preferences. Innovative approaches, such as telehealth interventions, wearable devices for activity monitoring, and integrative therapies, are being explored to enhance accessibility and effectiveness of fatigue management interventions. Collaborative efforts between researchers, healthcare providers, and survivors will continue to drive progress in identifying novel treatments and supportive care strategies to alleviate cancer-related fatigue and enhance survivorship outcomes.

Emerging Research on Fatigue

While considerable progress has been made

in understanding and managing CRF, emerging research is shedding new light on its underlying mechanisms, risk factors, and treatment approaches.

Advancements in Understanding CRF:

Emerging research on CRF is uncovering the multifactorial nature of this symptom, involving intricate interactions between biological, psychological, and social factors. While the exact mechanisms underlying CRF remain incompletely understood, recent studies suggest contributions from inflammation, alterations in neurotransmitter pathways, disruptions in circadian rhythms, and dysregulation of the hypothalamic-pituitary-adrenal axis.

Moreover, psychosocial factors such as stress, anxiety, depression, sleep disturbances, and poor coping strategies are increasingly recognized as important contributors to CRF. Social determinants of health, including socioeconomic status, social support networks, and access to healthcare resources, also play a significant role in shaping individuals' experiences of fatigue during and after cancer treatment.

Identifying Risk Factors and Predictors:

Emerging research is focused on identifying risk factors and predictors of CRF to better understand who is most vulnerable to developing this symptom and why. Studies have identified a variety of factors associated with increased risk of CRF, including older age, female gender, higher disease burden, comorbidities, treatment-related toxicities, genetic predisposition, and psychosocial distress.

Additionally, emerging evidence suggests that pre-existing conditions such as obesity, sedentary lifestyle, poor sleep quality, and psychological comorbidities may predispose individuals to develop CRF before cancer diagnosis or exacerbate fatigue during treatment. Understanding these risk factors and their interplay can inform targeted interventions to prevent or mitigate CRF and improve outcomes for cancer patients and survivors.

Innovations in Treatment and Management:

Innovative approaches to CRF treatment and management are being explored to address the diverse needs and preferences of cancer patients and survivors. While conventional interventions such as pharmacotherapy, exercise, and psychosocial support remain cornerstone strategies for managing CRF, emerging research is investigating novel therapies and integrative approaches to enhance fatigue relief and promote well-being.

For example, targeted pharmacological agents, including psychostimulants, cytokine modulators, and hormonal therapies, are being evaluated for their efficacy in alleviating CRF symptoms by targeting specific biological pathways implicated in fatigue. Furthermore, non-pharmacological interventions such as mindfulness-based stress reduction, acupuncture, yoga, massage therapy, and music therapy are gaining attention for their potential to improve fatigue-related outcomes and enhance overall quality of life.

Additionally, advances in technology, including mobile health applications, wearable devices, and telehealth platforms, offer innovative ways to deliver fatigue management interventions remotely, enhance patient engagement, and facilitate self-monitoring and self-management of symptoms. These digital health tools provide opportunities for personalized, real-time support and guidance, empowering patients to actively participate in their own care and optimize fatigue management outcomes.

Patient-Centered Approaches to Fatigue Management

Patient-centered approaches to fatigue management in cancer care prioritize the individual needs, preferences, and experiences of patients, empowering them to actively participate in their own care and decision-making process. Recognizing that cancer-related fatigue (CRF) is a complex and subjective symptom that affects each patient differently, these approaches aim to tailor interventions to address the unique challenges and goals of each individual.

Principles of Patient-Centered Fatigue Management:

1. Holistic Assessment:

- Patient-centered fatigue management begins with a comprehensive assessment of the patient's physical, emotional, and social well-being, as well as their values, preferences, and priorities. This holistic approach considers the full range of factors contributing to fatigue, including medical history, cancer treatment, comorbidities, psychosocial stressors, and lifestyle factors.

2. Shared Decision-Making:

- Shared decision-making is a core principle of patient-centered care that involves active collaboration between patients and healthcare providers in treatment planning and decision-making. In the context of fatigue management, patients are encouraged to share their concerns, preferences, and treatment goals with their healthcare team, and together, they explore various options and make informed decisions based on the best available evidence and the patient's values and preferences.

3. Individualized Interventions:

- Patient-centered fatigue management recognizes that there is no one-size-fits-all approach to addressing CRF. Instead, interventions are tailored to meet the unique needs, preferences, and circumstances of each patient. This may involve a combination of pharmacological and non-pharmacological strategies, including medication management, exercise, nutrition counseling, stress reduction techniques, psychosocial support, and complementary therapies.

4. Empowerment and Education:

- Patient empowerment and education are essential components of patient-centered fatigue management. Patients are provided with information, resources, and skills to actively participate in their own care, make informed decisions, and self-manage their symptoms. Healthcare providers serve as partners and facilitators in this process, offering guidance, support, and encouragement to empower patients to take control of their fatigue and overall well-being.

Benefits of Patient-Centered Fatigue Management:

1. Improved Symptom Relief:

- Patient-centered fatigue management has been shown to improve symptom relief and quality of life for cancer patients and survivors. By addressing the underlying factors contributing to fatigue and tailoring interventions to meet the individual needs of each patient, healthcare providers can optimize treatment outcomes and enhance patient satisfaction and well-being.

2. Enhanced Treatment Adherence:

- Patient-centered approaches to fatigue management promote treatment adherence by engaging patients as active participants in their own care. When patients feel heard, respected, and involved in decision-making, they are more likely to adhere to treatment recommendations and engage in self-management strategies to alleviate their symptoms.

3. Greater Patient Satisfaction:

- Patient-centered care fosters greater patient satisfaction and trust in the healthcare system. When patients feel valued, respected, and supported by their healthcare providers, they are more satisfied with their care experiences and more likely to have positive outcomes. Patient-centered approaches to fatigue management promote a collaborative and respectful relationship between patients and providers, leading to improved communication, trust, and satisfaction.

Strategies for Integrating Patient-Centered Approaches into Clinical Practice:

1. Establishing Open Communication:

- Establishing open, honest, and empathetic communication with patients is essential for patient-centered fatigue management. Healthcare providers should create a safe and supportive environment where patients feel comfortable expressing their concerns, asking questions, and actively participating in decision-making.

2. Individualized Assessment and Planning:

- Conducting a thorough assessment of each patient's fatigue symptoms, contributing factors, and treatment goals is essential for developing individualized care plans. Healthcare providers should collaborate with patients to identify their unique needs, preferences, and priorities and tailor interventions accordingly.

3. Educating and Empowering Patients:

- Educating patients about the causes and management of fatigue, as well as empowering them with skills and resources to self-manage their symptoms, is key to patient-centered care. Healthcare providers should provide clear, accessible information to patients and involve them in developing personalized self-management strategies.

4. Promoting Shared Decision-Making:

- Promoting shared decision-making involves actively involving patients in treatment planning and decision-making processes. Healthcare providers should engage patients in discussions about treatment options, risks, benefits, and alternatives, and support them in making informed decisions that align with their values, preferences, and goals.

5. Providing Ongoing Support and Follow-Up:

- Providing ongoing support and follow-up is

essential for maintaining patient engagement and addressing evolving needs throughout the cancer journey. Healthcare providers should regularly monitor patients' fatigue symptoms, treatment responses, and psychosocial well-being, and adjust interventions as needed to optimize outcomes and promote patient-centered care.

Areas for Future Exploration and Improvement

As our understanding of cancer-related fatigue (CRF) evolves and new challenges emerge, it is essential to explore areas for future exploration and improvement to enhance the quality of care and well-being of cancer patients and survivors.

1. Precision Medicine and Personalized Interventions:
   - Future research should focus on advancing precision medicine approaches to CRF management, tailoring interventions to the individual characteristics, preferences, and needs of patients. This includes identifying biomarkers, genetic markers, and psychosocial factors that predict treatment response and designing personalized interventions that address the specific underlying mechanisms driving fatigue in each patient.

2. Biopsychosocial Models of Care:
   - Integrating biopsychosocial models of care into CRF management can provide a comprehensive

framework for addressing the multifactorial nature of fatigue. Future research should explore the interactions between biological, psychological, and social factors contributing to CRF and develop integrated interventions that target these factors simultaneously to optimize treatment outcomes and enhance patient well-being.

3. Digital Health Technologies:

- The integration of digital health technologies, including mobile applications, wearable devices, and telehealth platforms, offers innovative opportunities to enhance CRF management and support patient self-management. Future research should explore the feasibility, effectiveness, and acceptability of digital health interventions for monitoring symptoms, delivering interventions, promoting adherence, and facilitating communication between patients and providers.

4. Longitudinal Studies and Survivorship Research:

- Longitudinal studies and survivorship research are essential for understanding the long-term trajectories of CRF, identifying risk factors for persistent fatigue, and exploring the impact of fatigue on survivors' quality of life and health outcomes. Future research should prioritize longitudinal studies that follow patients from diagnosis through survivorship, examining the dynamic interplay between fatigue, treatment effects, comorbidities, psychosocial factors, and health-related outcomes over time.

5. Cultural and Linguistic Considerations:
-   Addressing cultural and linguistic considerations is critical for ensuring equitable access to CRF management and support services for diverse populations. Future research should explore cultural factors influencing the experience and expression of fatigue, develop culturally tailored interventions and educational materials, and promote culturally competent care to meet the unique needs of patients from diverse backgrounds.

6. Interdisciplinary Collaboration and Care Coordination:
-   Interdisciplinary collaboration and care coordination are essential for delivering comprehensive and coordinated care to cancer patients and survivors. Future research should focus on fostering partnerships between oncologists, primary care providers, nurses, psychologists, rehabilitation specialists, and other healthcare professionals to integrate CRF management into routine cancer care and survivorship programs.

7. Patient and Caregiver Engagement:
- Engaging patients and caregivers as partners in research, care delivery, and advocacy is essential for ensuring that CRF management initiatives are patient-centered and responsive to the needs and priorities of those affected by cancer. Future research should involve patients and caregivers in the design, implementation, and evaluation

of interventions, prioritize their perspectives and experiences, and empower them to advocate for improved CRF management and support services.

HOLISTIC APPROACHES TO WELLNESS FOR CANCER SURVIVORS

Holistic approaches to wellness for cancer survivors emphasize the interconnectedness of the body, mind, and spirit, recognizing that optimal health and well-being require attention to all aspects of the individual. These approaches go beyond treating symptoms and diseases to promote overall wellness and quality of life by addressing physical, emotional, social, and spiritual needs.

Principles of Holistic Wellness for Cancer Survivors:

1. Comprehensive Assessment:
   - Holistic wellness for cancer survivors begins with a comprehensive assessment of the individual's physical health, emotional well-being, social support networks, lifestyle behaviors, and spiritual beliefs and practices. This assessment provides a holistic understanding of the survivor's needs, preferences, strengths, and challenges, guiding the development of personalized care plans.

2. Individualized Care Plans:
   - Holistic wellness approaches recognize that each survivor is unique and requires individualized care plans tailored to their specific needs, preferences, and goals. Care plans may include a combination

of conventional medical treatments, integrative therapies, lifestyle interventions, psychosocial support, and spiritual practices, tailored to meet the survivor's holistic needs and promote optimal well-being.

3. Multidisciplinary Collaboration:

- Holistic wellness for cancer survivors involves collaboration among multidisciplinary healthcare providers, including oncologists, primary care physicians, nurses, psychologists, nutritionists, physical therapists, and spiritual counselors. By working together as a team, healthcare providers can address the diverse needs of survivors and provide comprehensive care that addresses all aspects of their health and well-being.

4. Empowerment and Self-Management:

- Holistic wellness empowers survivors to take an active role in their own care and self-management, providing them with the knowledge, skills, and resources to make informed decisions and engage in behaviors that promote health and well-being. By empowering survivors to participate in their own care, holistic approaches foster a sense of agency, self-efficacy, and resilience.

Benefits of Holistic Wellness for Cancer Survivors:

1. Improved Physical Health:

- Holistic approaches to wellness promote improved physical health by addressing the physical consequences of cancer and its treatment, such as fatigue, pain, neuropathy, lymphedema, and hormonal imbalances. Integrative therapies such as acupuncture, massage therapy, yoga, and exercise can help alleviate symptoms, improve function, and enhance overall physical well-being.

2. Enhanced Emotional Well-Being:
- Holistic wellness supports survivors' emotional well-being by addressing the psychological impact of cancer, such as anxiety, depression, fear of recurrence, and existential distress. Psychosocial interventions such as counseling, support groups, mindfulness meditation, and expressive arts therapy can help survivors cope with emotional challenges, enhance coping skills, and foster emotional resilience.

3. Improved Quality of Life:
- By addressing the physical, emotional, social, and spiritual dimensions of health, holistic wellness approaches contribute to improved quality of life for cancer survivors. These approaches help survivors live more fully, with greater vitality, purpose, and meaning, even in the face of cancer-related challenges and uncertainties.

4. Enhanced Survivorship Experience:
- Holistic wellness enhances the survivorship experience by promoting a sense of wholeness, connection, and empowerment. By addressing survivors' holistic needs and promoting self-care, self-awareness, and self-compassion, holistic

approaches foster a positive survivorship narrative that emphasizes resilience, growth, and post-traumatic growth.

Strategies for Integrating Holistic Wellness into Survivorship Care:

1. Comprehensive Survivorship Care Plans:
   - Survivorship care plans should include comprehensive assessments of survivors' holistic needs and preferences, as well as individualized care plans that address physical, emotional, social, and spiritual aspects of wellness. These care plans should be developed collaboratively with survivors and their healthcare providers, incorporating input from multidisciplinary team members as needed.

2. Access to Integrative Therapies:
   - Survivorship programs should provide survivors with access to a range of integrative therapies and supportive care services that address their holistic needs. These may include acupuncture, massage therapy, yoga, meditation, art therapy, music therapy, nutrition counseling, and exercise programs, offered in conjunction with conventional medical treatments.

3. Psychosocial Support and Counseling:
   - Psychosocial support services, including individual counseling, support groups, and peer mentoring programs, should be readily available to survivors to help them cope with emotional challenges, enhance resilience, and foster social

connection. These services should be tailored to meet survivors' diverse needs and preferences and provide culturally competent care.

4. Education and Empowerment:

- Survivorship programs should provide survivors with education, resources, and skills to promote self-care, self-management, and self-advocacy. This may include information on healthy lifestyle behaviors, stress management techniques, coping strategies, survivorship resources, and community support services, delivered through a variety of formats and modalities.

5. Spiritual Care and Support:

- Spiritual care and support should be integrated into survivorship programs to address survivors' spiritual needs, beliefs, and practices. This may include providing opportunities for spiritual reflection, prayer, meditation, ritual, and connection with spiritual communities and providers. Spiritual counselors or chaplains trained in providing spiritual care to individuals affected by cancer can offer support, guidance, and resources to help survivors navigate spiritual questions, existential concerns, and the search for meaning and purpose in their survivorship journey.

6. Promotion of Healthy Lifestyle Behaviors:

- Survivorship programs should promote healthy lifestyle behaviors that support survivors' overall well-being, including regular physical activity, balanced nutrition, adequate sleep, stress management, and avoidance of tobacco and excessive alcohol consumption. Education, resources, and support should be provided to help survivors adopt and maintain healthy habits that contribute to long-term health and well-being.

7. Long-Term Follow-Up and Support:

- Holistic wellness should be integrated into long-term follow-up care for cancer survivors, with ongoing monitoring of survivors' holistic needs, treatment effects, and quality of life. Survivorship programs should provide continuous support and resources to survivors as they navigate the challenges and transitions of survivorship, ensuring that they feel supported and empowered to thrive in their post-treatment lives.

ABOUT THE AUTHOR

Dr. Bhratri Bhushan

Dr. Bhratri Bhushan is a consultant medical oncologist and hematologist. He has a rich academic and research background, having published more than two hundred books 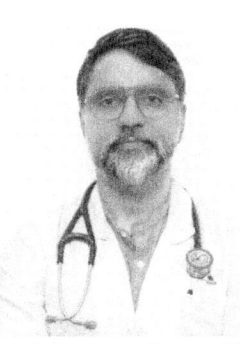 on the subjects of oncology and internal medicine. His scholarly contributions have been featured in renowned journals of medical literature. For a comprehensive collection of his works, please visit his AuthorCentral page at www.amazon.com/author/bhratribhushan